KN

AND

DISABILITY

RENE CAILLIET, M.D.

Chairman and Professor
Department of Rehabilitative Medicine
University of Southern California School of Medicine
Los Angeles, California

F. A. DAVIS COMPANY *Philadelphia*

Also by Rene Cailliet:

FOOT AND ANKLE PAIN
HAND PAIN AND IMPAIRMENT
LOW BACK PAIN SYNDROME
NECK AND ARM PAIN
SHOULDER PAIN
SOFT TISSUE PAIN AND DISABILITY

Preface

The knee of the human biped is subjected daily from birth to senility to numerous stresses, injuries, and diseases, and it places high in percentage of patients disabled from musculoskeletal impairment in comparison with lumbrosacral pain, neck and shoulder pain, foot pain, and hand dysfunction. As stated in the introduction of Chapter One, the knee is probably the most complicated joint in the human body.

Therefore, this monograph is offered in an effort to acquaint the student, intern, resident, family practitioner, and nonorthopedist with basic knee conditions they may see, often in the early phase of pain or disability. As in the previous CAILLIET PAIN SERIES, functional anatomy is stressed and illustrations are schematic for simplification and economy.

In order to maintain the small size of this addition to the series, neither exhaustive presentations of the subjects that are discussed in this book nor *all* knee conditions can be included. New forms of treatment emerge daily, such as the total knee replacement, and new concepts of disease and disability become clarified by continuing research and clinical experience. Only constant study can keep the practicing physician and therapist abreast of advancing scientific knowledge.

It is hoped this book will lead to earlier recognition of knee conditions, better evaluation, increased physiological treatment, and earlier referral for more definitive and specialized treatment when so recognized.

RENE CAILLIET, M.D.

Table of Contents

Illustrations

CHAPTER 1

Structural Anatomy

The knee joint is probably the most complicated joint in the human body. It is intricate because its function is related to its gross bony anatomy, integrated muscular activity, and precise restrictive ligamentous structures. Its articular surfaces frequently are exposed to stresses and strains. Because of the knee's complexity and frequency to pain, a thorough knowledge of functional anatomy is mandatory for a meaningful examination, proper evaluation of symptoms and findings, and a physiological basis for treatment.

OSSEOUS COMPONENTS

The joint is formed by the distal end of the femur and the proximal end of the tibia with interposed menisci, which give symmetry to the joint and aid in lubrication. Ligaments and muscles surround the joint. Motion is basically that of flexion and extension with minimal rotatory motion. The human knee, unlike that of lower primates, is capable of full extension (0°) and greater than 90° flexion. Slight abduction and adduction are physiologically possible with the tibia fully extended upon the femur.

The joint surface of the distal femur has two surfaces (Fig. 1): anteriorly the femoral patellar and inferiorly the tibial. The patellar surface is saddle shaped and is asymmetrical, with the lateral face larger and more convex than the medial plate. Upon this surface glides the patella, an integral part of the knee extensor mechanism.

The tibial surface of the femur viewed laterally is flattened in its anterior surface and curved on its posterior lateral aspect. The inferior surface of the femur is formed by two condyles

1

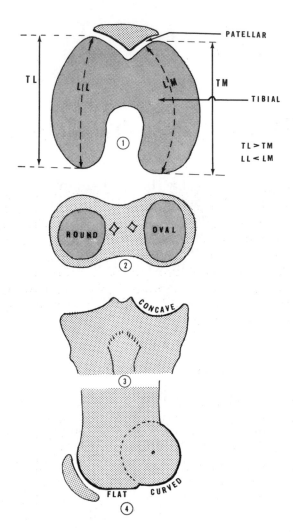

FIGURE 1. Knee joint surfaces. *1*, Femoral condyle surfaces of the right knee. *TL*, Anteroposterior length of the lateral condyle; *TM*, Length of the medial condyle. The length of the medial condyle, *LM*, is greater than the length of the lateral condyle, *LL*, because of its curved surface. *2*, Superior surface of the right tibia. The lateral articular surface is rounded and the medial articular surface is oval. *3*, The medial tibial articular surface is deeper and more concave than is the lateral. *4*, Side view of the femur showing the flat anterior surface and the curved posterior surface. The two articulations are illustrated in *1*: the patellar in which the patella articulates with the anterior femur and the tibial then glides upon the tibia.

separated by a deep U-shaped notch, the intercondylar fossa. This fossa is deep and wide, equal in size to that of a thumb. The medial femoral condyle has a smaller transverse diameter (TM in Fig. 1) but a longer longitudinal diameter (LM in Fig. 1) because of its curved direction. These condylar surfaces correspond to similiar articular surfaces of the opposing tibial condyles.

The tibial plateau has two articular surfaces (see Fig. 1). Viewed in an anteroposterior direction, the medial surface is oval, deeper, and more concave than its lateral and rounder counterpart. The two surfaces arch upward towards each other and are separated by two bony spines, the eminentia intercondylaris (Fig. 2).

All articular surfaces of the femoral condyles, the tibial condyles, and the dorsal aspect of the patella are covered by cartilage with a thickness of 3 to 4 mm.

The joint capsule is large, permitting injection of 30 to 40 cc. of air before causing tension. The capsule attaches to the femur near the margins of the articular cartilage at the site of the epicondyles. It is attached upon the tibia just distal to the attachment of the collateral ligaments. In the joint the synovial membrane passes anteriorly to the cruciate ligament, thus making the cruciate ligaments *inter*articular but *extra*capsular (Fig. 3).

FIGURE 2.   Superficial landmarks of the knee bones. *Above,* femur; *Below,* tibia.

3

FIGURE 3.   Synovial capsule. The knee joint capsule is large and shallow and can hold up to 40 cc. of air without tension. *1*, Anteriorly it ascends to two finger breadths above the patella. *2*, Posteriorly it ascends to the origin of the gastrocnemius muscle. *3*, Laterally it attaches to the femur at the junction of the condylar cartilage at the epicondylar level. *4*, Inferiorly it attaches upon the tibia a quarter inch below the articular margin at the attachment of the collateral ligament. *5*, The cruciate ligaments invaginate the capsule; thus they are extracapsular.

4

The asymmetry of the relationship of the femoral condyles to the tibial condyles is compensated by the interposed menisci. These are curved, wedged, fibrocartilaginous structures that lie between the opposing articular surfaces. They are connected to each other and to the joint capsule. These menisci assist in distributing the pressure between the femur and the tibia, increase the elasticity of the joint, and assist in its lubrication.

The medial meniscus is approximately 10 mm. wide with its posterior horn wider than the middle portion (Fig. 4). The medial meniscus has a wider curve than the lateral meniscus. Its anterior horn connects to the anterior ridge of the tibia by fibrous ligamentous tissue and to the ventral intercondylar spine. It often connects with the anterior cruciate ligament. By way of the ligamentous transversus it connects to the anterior horn of the lateral meniscus. Around its outer periphery it is firmly connected to the joint capsule and the medial collateral ligament.

Posteriorly the medial meniscus connects to a fibrous thickening of the capsule and is connected to the tendinous portion of the semimembranous muscle.

The lateral meniscus has a width of 12 to 13 mm. Its curvature is greater than the medial meniscus, causing it to resemble a

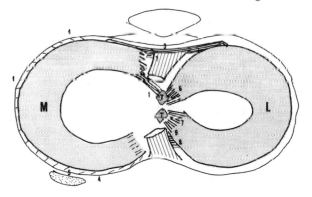

FIGURE 4. Attachments of the menisci. Right tibial plateau viewed from above. 1, Fibrous attachment of the medial meniscus, M, to outer ridge of the tibial tubercle, T. 2, Connection to the anterior cruciate ligament and 3, to the anterior horn of the lateral meniscus, L, via the ligamentous transversus. 4, The medial meniscus is attached around its entire periphery to the capsule and 5, posteriorly to the semimembranosus muscle tendon. The lateral meniscus has both its 6, anterior and 7, posterior horns attached to the eminentia intercondylaris, T, by a fibrous connection, 8, to the posterior cruciate ligament. 9, A fibrous band attaches superiorly into the fossa intercondylaris of the femur.

closed ring. Both the anterior and posterior horns of the lateral meniscus insert directly into the eminentia intercondylaris and by a fibrous connection to the posterior cruciate ligament, the ligamentous menisci fibularis. Most of the posterior horn inserts into the femur through the fossa intercondylaris and via a strong fasciculus that proceeds upward and medially. This is known as the ligament of Wrisberg and often blends with the posterior cruciate ligament.

The lateral meniscus has very loose connections to the lateral capsule and its posterior horn has the popliteus tendon sheath interposed between it and the capsule. A synovial pouch (recessus inferior) may occur between the meniscus and the capsule. Its outer wall contains the popliteus tendon; this compartment is called the sheath of the popliteus tendon. The lateral meniscus has great mobility because of its bony connection centrally with the spines and little or no lateral capsular connection.

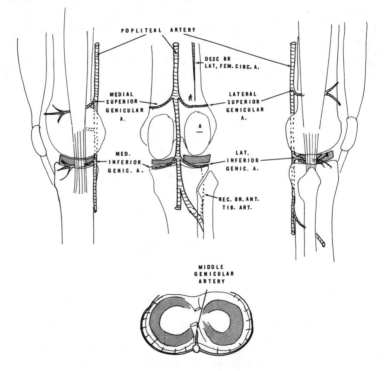

FIGURE 5. Blood supply of the knee joint. The popliteal artery has five branches in the area of the knee joint.

6

BLOOD SUPPLY

The popliteal artery, a continuation of the femoral artery, has five branches in the area of the knee joint (Fig. 5): the medial and lateral superior geniculars, the middle genicular, and the medial and lateral inferior geniculars.

The superior geniculars curve around the femoral condyles proximal to the epicondyles and form a plexus in the suprapatellar area. The inferior genicular branches course around the margin of the tibial plateau passing under the collateral ligaments. The middle genicular arises from the posterior portion of the popliteal artery, pierces the popliteal ligament, and sends three branches: the middle follows the anterior cruciate ligament and the medial and lateral branches enter the perimeniscal connective tissue zone (Fig. 6).

The middle and inferior genicular branches supply the menisci which are mostly avascular. Only the outer one third and the central portion of the meniscus have any significant blood supply.

The superior genicular plexus is joined by the descending branch of the lateral femoral circumflex artery and the inferior genicular plexus is joined by the recurrent branch of the anterior tibial artery.

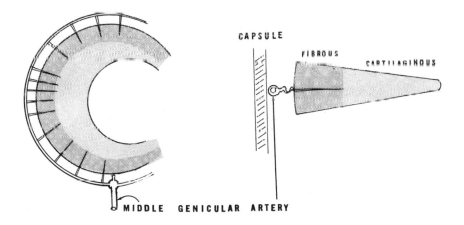

FIGURE 6. Intrinsic circulation of the menisci. The middle genicular artery sends branches around the loose connective tissue of the perimeniscal zone under the capsule. Nonanastomatic small vessels, tortuous to permit movement, enter the fibrous zone (outer third) of the meniscus. They are more numerous in the central area of the meniscus. The inner third (cartilaginous zone) is avascular.

LIGAMENTS

The bony configuration of the knee joint contributes little to the stability and integrity of the joint. Strength is dependent upon the integrity of the muscles and secondarily upon the ligaments. The ligaments comprising the joint structure are the cruciates, the collaterals, and the joint capsule.

FIGURE 7.   Cruciate ligaments. *1*, Viewed from posterior aspect of right knee with knee bent; *2*, Superior view of tibial plateau; *3*, Posterior view of extended right knee; *4*, Side view of knee.

A = Anterior ligaments
P = Posterior ligaments
M = Medial ligaments
L = Lateral ligaments

Cruciate

The paired cruciate ligaments are named according to their tibial attachments. The anterior ligament proceeds superiorly and posteriorly from its anterior medial tibial attachment to attach to the medial aspect of the lateral femoral condyle (Fig. 7) and the posterior cruciate arises from the back of the tibia and extends forward, upward, and inward to attach to the medial femoral condyle. The cruciate ligaments prevent shear motion of the knee joint and act to guide the flexion-rotation of the knee joint. The posterior cruciate ligament prevents excessive *internal* rotation of the tibia upon the femur. The anterior cruciate prevents abnormal *external* rotation.

By its attachment and direction (Fig. 8), the anterior cruciate ligament stabilizes the knee in extension and prevents hyperextension. The posterior cruciate aids normal knee flexion by acting as a drag during the primary glide.

Capsular and Collateral

The capsular ligaments and collateral ligaments stabilize the joint by guiding as well as restricting joint motion. The collateral ligaments are essentially a selective thickening of the fibrous capsule of the joint. They can be divided into a medial and lateral portion, each having specific characteristics (Fig. 9).

Medial Capsular. The medial capsular ligaments divide into deep and superficial sections. The deep section in turn is divisible into three portions: the anterior, middle, and posterior ligaments (Fig. 10). The anterior portion has parallel fibers that cover the anterior aspect of the joint, extend anteriorly into the extension mechanism, and attach loosely to the medial meniscus. These fibers are slightly relaxed during knee extension but become taut during flexion (Fig. 11). The posterior fibers are oblique (fanned), thin, and indistinct. They continue posteriorly to aid in the formation of the posterior popliteal capsule. They are attached to the posterior medial aspect of the medial meniscus and blend with the semimembranosus muscle.

The middle third of the deep medial capsular ligament has more distinct fibers and comprises a superior and inferior division (Fig. 12). The superior is thicker and fixes the medial meniscus to the femur (the meniscofemoral segment) while the inferior is looser (meniscotibial) and permits the tibia to move upon the meniscus.

9

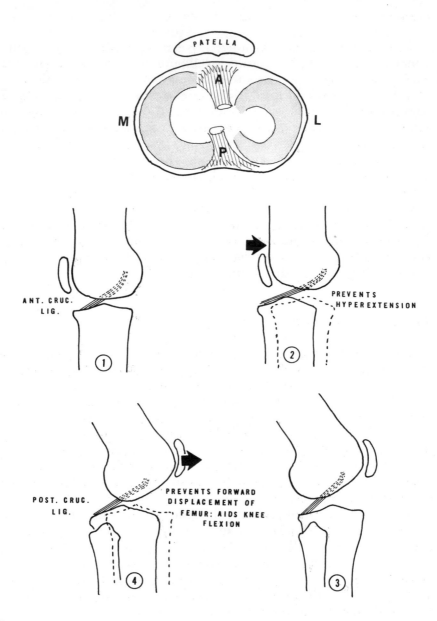

FIGURE 8. Function and restriction imposed upon cruciate ligaments. *Above*, Superior view of the point of attachment and direction of the cruciates. Right knee medial aspect: *1*, Direction of anterior cruciate and *2*, method of preventing hyperextension of the knee. Right knee lateral aspect: *3*, The posterior cruciate ligament and *4*, manner in which it prevents forward displacement of the femur upon the tibia. By acting as a drag force it aids in normal knee flexion.

Medial Collateral. The medial collateral ligament is principally the superficial medial ligament. It attaches superiorly to the femoral medial epicondyle and inferiorly upon the tibia just below the level of the articular cartilage. The anterior fibers are parallel and distinct. The posterior fibers converge into oblique fibers that are thinner and less distinct and that blend into the deep posterior capsular ligaments and into the semimembranous muscle tendon. Fibers from the posterior fibers attach to the medial meniscus. Numerous bursa (usually five) are interposed between the deep middle capsular ligament and the superficial collateral ligament (see Fig. 12).

Lateral Capsular. The fibular collateral ligament passes from

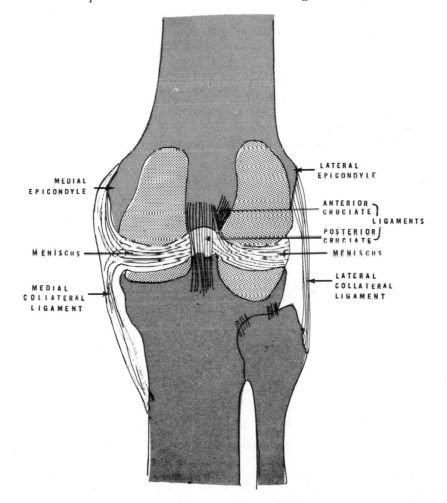

FIGURE 9. Capsular and collateral ligaments.

11

the lateral epicondyle of the femur to the head of the fibula (Fig. 13) where it is surrounded by the divided tendons of the biceps. The popliteus tendon passes beneath the fibular (lateral) ligament as it passes to attach to the lateral epicondyle of the femur. The underlying capsule thickens in its extension from the lateral femoral condyle to the fibular head to form a short fibular collateral ligament called the arcuate ligament.

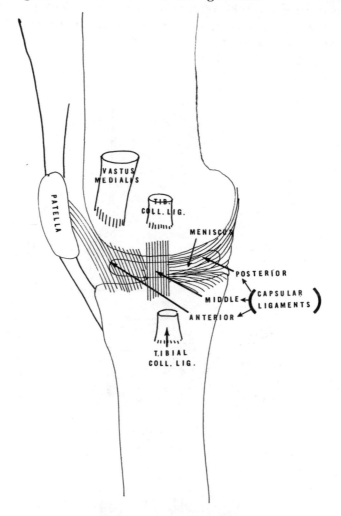

FIGURE 10. Medial (tibial) superficial collateral ligament. The three segments of the capsular ligament are shown: the parallel fibers of the anterior portion, the middle vertical, and the fanned indistinct posterior fibers. The superficial collateral ligament attaches just superior to the femoral medial epicondyle and to the tibia just below the articular cartilage and posterior to a point above the insertion of the semimembranous tendon.

The posterior border of the arcuate lies over the popliteal fascia, covering it and attached firmly to it. The arcuate is also firmly attached to the posterior arch of the lateral meniscus. The upper fibers of the popliteus muscle attach to the arcuate ligament and the lateral meniscus (see Fig. 13). The peroneal nerve passes the neck of the fibula behind the biceps tendon.

The posterior popliteal fossa of the knee joint is bounded superiorly by the semimembranosus and semitendinosus tendons and the biceps tendon and inferiorly by the two heads of the gastrocnemius muscle. The roof consists of the popliteal

ANTERIOR THIRD

POSTERIOR THIRD

FIGURE 11. Motion of medial ligaments during knee flexion. *1*, The anterior fibers are slightly slack during knee extension and *2*, taut during flexion. *3* and *4*, The opposite action of the posterior fibers.

13

fascia under which lie the popliteal artery, vein, and nerve. The popliteal nerve divides into the tibial and peroneal branches in the upper portion of the fossa with the peroneal branch passing over the lateral head of the gastrocnemius under the fascia.

FIGURE 12. Deep medial and superficial collateral ligamentous action. The middle segment of the deep medial capsular ligament is divided into *1*, a superior portion that fixes the medial meniscus to the femur during flexion and *2*, an inferior portion that is slack and permits the meniscus to move. Joint spaces called meniscofemoral and meniscotibial are arbitrarily formed. *3* and *4* show the relationship of a bursa to the superficial and deep medial ligaments.

14

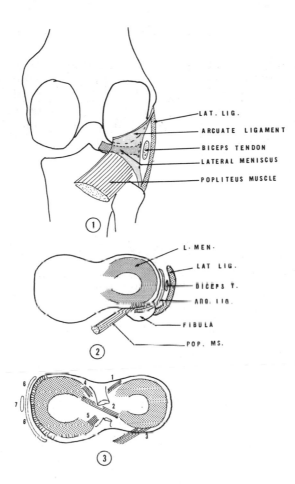

FIGURE 13. Lateral ligaments of knee. *1*, The deep part of the lateral ligament attaches from the femoral epicondyle to the styloid process and tibial
border of the fibular head. The posterior border lying across the popliteus
muscle forms the arcuate ligament. The arcuate ligament attaches firmly to the
posterior horn of the lateral ligament. Between the lateral ligament attachment
and the arcuate ligament pass the tendon of the biceps femoris muscle. *2*, The
popliteus muscle emerges beneath the arcuate ligament to insert medioposte-
riorly on the tibia. The muscle originates partly from the arcuate ligament
margin and from the posterior aspect of the meniscus. When the knee flexes
this muscle probably pulls the meniscus and simultaneously externally rotates
itself, thus protecting the meniscus. *3*, Attachment of menisci. The lateral
menisci is attached at both horns to the tibia, *1–2*, with *2* crossing over from the
posterior horn of the lateral meniscus to the anterior horn of the medial
meniscus and the femoral attachment of the anterior cruciate ligament. There
are fibrous bands, *1–4*, that connect anterior horns of both menisci to the
femoral attachments of the anterior cruciate. The medial meniscus is attached
by its anterior and posterior horns with fibrous bands, *4–5*, and along the
entire circumference of the capsule, *6*, and the superficial medial ligament, *7*.

15

The knee is powerfully motored and stabilized by muscles that cross the joint from origin above the hip joint, from the entire femoral shaft, and from origin above the knee of lower leg muscles. For convenience, muscle groups can be classified as anterior (knee *extensor*), posterior (knee *flexors*), medial (*adductors*), and lateral (*abductors*). Both abductors and adductors are also rotators and stabilizers.

Extensors

The major muscle of the extensor group is the quadriceps femoris, comprising four heads: the rectus femoris and three vasti named the medialis, lateralis, and intermedius. The rectus originates from the anterior inferior iliac spine; thus, it crosses the hip joint and influences hip motion. The vasti arise from the shaft of the femur. All four muscles converge into a common tendon that crosses the knee joint and attaches to the tibial tuberosity (Fig. 14) via the patella.

The patella (Fig. 15), long considered a sesamoid bone, provides with the femur a gliding surface that minimizes frictional attrition and provides mechanical leverage (Figs. 16 and 17). The quadriceps femoris tendon comprises three lamina: the superficial layer from the rectus, the middle layer from tendons of the vasti lateralis and medialis, and a deep layer from the vastus intermedius. Some of the tendon fibers pass over (anterior to) the patella; some attach to the superior and some to the lateral borders of the patella. Fibers from the lateral and medial aspects of the patella fan out to either side to insert into the femoral condyles (see Fig. 15) and some fibers pass to the capsular and collateral ligaments to attach to the menisci (see Fig. 16).

Superficial to the quadriceps in the anterior aspect of the thigh is the sartorius muscle. This ribbonlike muscle spirals across the thigh from its origin at the anterosuperior spine to the anterosuperior-medial portion of the tibia (Fig. 18). Although there are other thigh muscles (the lateral and medial groups: the adductors and abductors), they function mostly upon the hip joint and will not be detailed here. Reference to standard texts is encouraged.

The nerve supply of the quadriceps group is the femoral nerve, which is formed by the anterior primary division of L_{2-4}. Its sensory distribution is depicted in Figure 19. In addition to

16

motor function, the knee-jerk (deep tendon) reflex is dependent upon the integrity of this nerve and its roots.

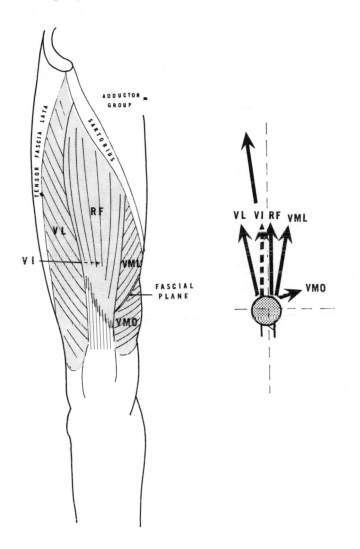

FIGURE 14. Quadriceps femoris: function of quadriceps mechanism. Each long component of the quadriceps group (*RF*, rectus femoris; *VL*, vastus lateralis; *VI*, vastus intermedius; *VM*, vastus medialis) can extend the knee fully. The vastus medialis oblique fibers, *VMO*, cannot extend the knee but apparently pulls the patella medially (right) and keeps it centered against lateral pull of the quadriceps, *arrows*. All long components pull equally throughout extension range with *VMO* exerting twice the force of contraction. The mechanics of the joint determine weakness (less efficiency) in the last 15° to 20°.

17

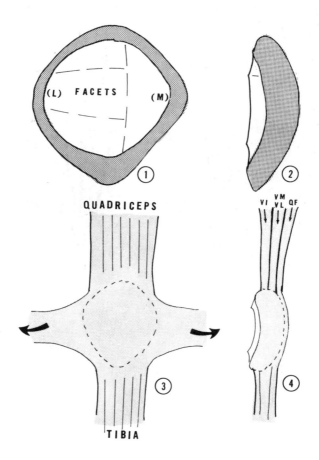

FIGURE 15. Patella. *1*, Ventral view showing the articular surfaces divided into three medial facets and a lateral facet that articulate with the femur. The lateral aspect is wider than the medial. The rough bone presents the surface upon which the patellar extensor mechanism attaches. *2*, Lateral view of the patella. *3*, The quadriceps attaches to the patella. Laterally and medially, *arrows*, fibers extend to attach to the femoral condyles and the capsulomeniscal tissues. *4*, The three layers of the tendinous insertion. The quadriceps, *QR*, covers the anterior aspect of the patella. The vasti medialis and lateralis, *VM* and *VL*, attach to the middle (superior and lateral) aspects of the patella and the vastus intermedius, *VI*, to the posterior (superior) margin.

18

The posterior thigh and leg muscles also cross the knee and act to flex and rotate the leg upon the femur. They can best be divided into the medial and lateral groups (Fig. 20). The medial group contains the semimembranosus and semitendinosus muscles, which, when the knee is flexed, internally rotate the lower leg upon the femur. The biceps femoris is the main lateral

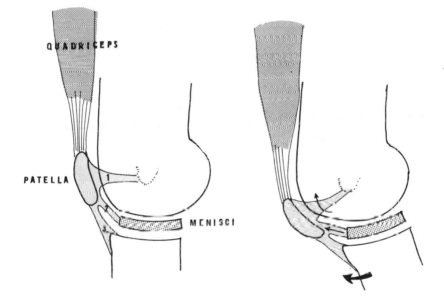

FIGURE 16. Quadriceps mechanism. The quadriceps extends over the anterior knee joint with three ligamentous extensions: *1*, the epicondylopatellar portion attaches to the epicondyle eminence of the femur and guides rotation of the patella; *2*, the meniscopatellar attaches to and pulls the meniscus forward during knee extension; and *3*, the infrapatellar tendon, which attaches to the tibial tubercle and extends the tibia upon the femur.

$$T = F \times M_{(A \text{ or } B)}$$

X – AXIS ROTATION
F – FORCE
M – ARM MOMENT

F = F

M > m ∴ T¹ > T²

$\overline{c}$ m F MUST·INCREASE 30%

FIGURE 17. Mechanical function of the patella. *Above,* Parallelograms of forces. When force is applied perpendicular to arm to rotate around axis, *X,* torque equals *F* times length of arm, M_A. With force applied oblique to arm, the moment becomes the distance from the force, *F,* to the axis, *X;* thus torque $T = F \times M_B$. *Below,* In the knee, the patella increases the arm moment from *m* to *M* and thus torque, T^1, is greater than T^2 with similar force, *F.* If the patella is not present, it has been calculated that a 30 percent increase in quadriceps strength is necessary to create equal torque. These forces are computed to knee rotation but disregard translation (gliding).

20

muscle of the hamstring group and, when the knee is flexed, it rotates the leg externally (Fig. 21).

The semitendinosus muscle originates from the ischial tuberosity (see Fig. 20), blending with the origin of the long head of the biceps femoris. After descending the medial aspect of the thigh, it crosses the knee joint and joins the sartorius and gracilis

FIGURE 18.   Sartorius muscle: tensor fascia lata. The sartorius muscle is a weak flexor of the knee and hip. The tensor fascia lata, which acts upon the knee, is considered to be a knee extensor but its primary function is abduction and stabilization of the hip.

21

muscles in a tendon, the pes anserinus, which flexes the knee (Fig. 22).

The semimembranosus arises from the ischial tuberosity lateral to the semitendinosus and descends the femur under the semitendinosus. It inserts by four tendons into the posteromedial side of the medial tibial condyle (Fig. 23) and sends

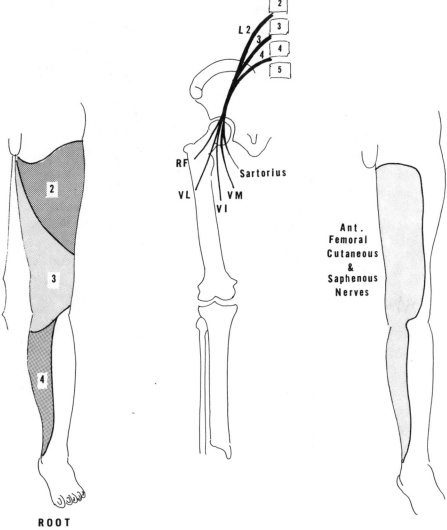

ROOT DERMATOMES

FIGURE 19. Distribution of the femoral nerve: its root formation. *Left,* Root dermatomes of the leg and thigh. *Center,* Formation of the nerve with anterior primary divisions of L $_2$, L $_3$, and L $_4$. *Right,* Cutaneous sensory distribution of the lower extremity.

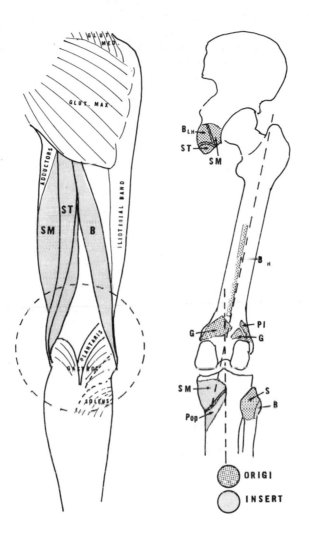

FIGURE 20.   Posterior thigh muscles: flexors. *Left*, The semimembranosus, *SM;* semitendinosus, *ST;* and the biceps femoris, *B*. The other muscles are labelled. *Right*, The origin and insertion of the posterior muscle groups.

B_{LH} = Biceps long head
B_{SH} = Biceps short head
B   = Biceps
S   = Sartorius
P1 = Plantaris
Pop = Popliteus
G   = Heads of gastrocnemius

fibers anteriorly to blend into the medial capsule and posteriorly to blend with the popliteal capsule. A deep fibrous branching attaches to the posterior horn of the medial meniscus and pulls the meniscus posteriorly when the semimembranosus flexes the knee.

The lateral flexor of the knee is primarily the biceps femoris muscle. The long head originates in the ischial tuberosity, descends the posterior thigh, and merges with the short head, which originates from the linea aspera of the femur. The long head forms a broad flat tendon 7 to 10 cm. above the level of the knee joint. It is joined on its undersurface at the fibular head to form a thick common tendon (Fig. 24).

The common biceps tendon passes downward and forward

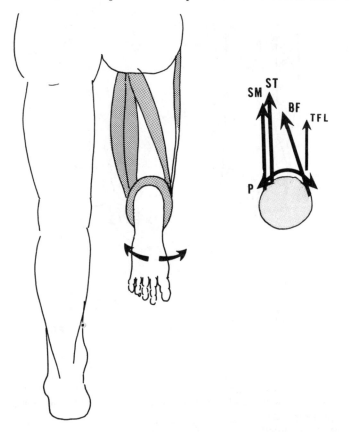

FIGURE 21. Rotators of the leg. When the knee is flexed the semimembranosus, *SM*, and the semitendinosus, *ST*, inwardly rotate the tibia. The biceps femoris, *BF*, and the tensor fascia lata, *TFL*, externally rotate the leg. The popliteus, *P*, originating laterally and inserting medially, internally rotates the leg upon the femur.

towards the knee joint. When it reaches the collateral ligament it splits into three layers: the superficial, middle, and deep.

The superficial layer forms three expansions: an anterior, middle, and posterior expansion. The anterior (Fig. 25) is thin, but strong, and fans out foward and down the lower leg. The middle expansion is thin and splits to surround the collateral ligament; these layers are separated from the ligament by bursae medially (inner), anteriorly, and laterally (outer). The posterior layer of the expansion is connected to the collateral ligament and to the joint capsule by a firm fibrous attachment. The deep layer bifurcates into a fibular and a tibial attachment (see Fig. 25) passing behind (medial to) the collateral ligament before attaching into the fibular head and the posterior aspect of the joint capsule.

The biceps femoris muscle functions to flex and to rotate externally the leg upon the femur when the knee is flexed (see Fig. 21). Passively pulling the superficial layer of the biceps

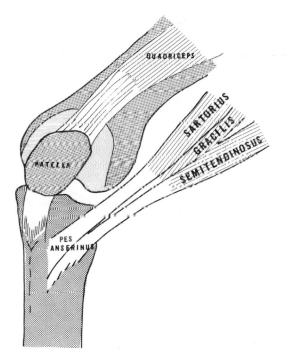

FIGURE 22. Pes anserinus. The medial insertion of the outer hamstring group forms a conjoined tendon of the semitendinosus with the sartorius and the gracilis muscles to form the pes anserinus. This tendon is separated from the underlying femoral condyle by a bursa.

insertion tendon flexes the knee and externally rotates the leg. As the knee flexes, the middle layer pulls upon the collateral ligament causing it to bow posteriorly and causing some slack in it. By its attachment of the deep portion to the joint capsule, as the knee flexes this expansion prevents impingement of the capsule between the tibia and the femur. This expansion is also

FIGURE 23.   Medial aspect of the posterior knee structure. *A,* The semi-membranosus muscle has four tendinous inserts. The major insert, *1,* extends to attach on the posterior aspect of the tibia and sends fibers into the popliteus. In its path there is an exterior branch that attaches to the posterior aspect of the medial meniscus, *2* and *3.* These tendons complete the posterior popliteal fossa and tense the capsule. *B,* The medial aspect of the knee with the insertion sites of the medial flexors. *C,* The semimembranosus flexes the knee and simultaneously pulls the meniscus backwards and rotates it with the tibia.

attached to the tensor (iliotibial band) and thus keeps the iliotibial band taut through knee flexion. As the biceps expansion bows the collateral ligament to maintain slack, it tightens the iliotibial band: this latter is most taut at 10° to 30° of flexion.

The flexor muscles receive their nerve supply from the sciatic nerve. After the sciatic nerve divides into its tibial and common peroneal nerve, the tibial nerve supplies the semimembranosus, semitendinosus, and the long head of the biceps; the short head of the biceps is supplied by the common peroneal branch.

FIGURE 24.   Biceps femoris tendon. The long head remains fleshy until about 10 cm. above the knee joint where it becomes a flat tendon. The short head remains fleshy until the fibular head. The common tendon then splits into three layers: S, superficial; M, middle; D, deep.

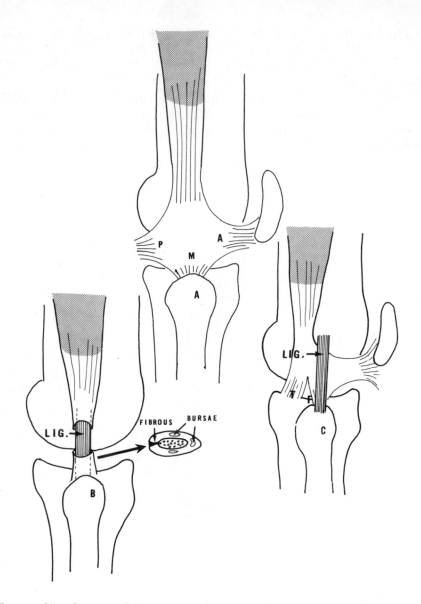

FIGURE 25.   Layers of the common biceps tendon. *A*, Superficial layer. The tendon divides into three expansions: *A*, anterior, which fans out to blend with the anterior crural fascia: middle, which extends to the collateral ligament at the fibular head; *P*, posterior, which blends with the fascia of the calf and lateral leg muscles. *B*, Middle layer. This is a thin layer which splits to envelop the lateral collateral ligament. The insert depicts the relationship of the bursae and the posterior fibrous attachment to the ligament. *C*, Deep layer. This layer bifurcates with one portion attaching to the fibular head, *F*, and the anterior half passing behind (medial to) the ligament and attaching to the tibia, *T*. Both attach to the knee joint capsule.

28

The popliteus muscle forms a part of the floor of the posterior knee fossa. It arises from the lateral epicondyle of the femur and runs posteromedially to attach to the posterior surface of the tibia. It rotates the leg internally upon the femur and is a weak knee flexor.

Gastrocnemius

The gastrocnemius muscles, essentially plantar flexors of the foot and ankle, by their origin above the knee joint have an effect on the knee joint. The gastrocnemius arises from two heads, medial and lateral, from the epicondyles of the femur. They quickly unite and descend the leg, joining the soleus muscle below the knee joint. The conjoined tendon ultimately attaches to the calcaneus.

When the leg is not weight bearing the gastrocnemius acts to flex the knee; when it is weight bearing the gastrocnemius *extends* the knee (Fig. 26). Without the quadriceps functioning the leg can be fully extended and can become a stable weight-bearing extremity. The foot, fixed to the floor, becomes the *origin* of the gastrocnemius which now can be considered to *insert* to the lower femur and upper tibia and pull these posteriorly, thus extending the knee. The knee joint now *locks* on its posterior capsule. At the hip joint the gluteus maximus extends the femur and weight bearing is now borne upon the anterior (hip joint capsule) Y ligament of Bigelow. Erect stance is now accomplished by ligamentous structures and minimal sporadic isometric contractions of the gastrocnemius and soleus muscles.

BURSAE

Bursae are normally located at sites of moving tissue to permit friction-free action and diminish attrition and inflammation of these contiguous tissues. There are 11 or more bursae in the region of the knee joint (Fig. 27). Three communicate with the knee joint: quadriceps (suprapatellar), popliteus, and the medial gastrocnemius. Three are related to the patella and the patellar tendon: prepatellar, superficial infrapatellar, and the deep infrapatellar. Two relate to the semimembranosus tendons: one, which communicates with the gastrocnemius bursa and/or the knee joint, lies between the semimembranosus tendons and the gastrocnemius tendon, and the other lies between the semimembranosus tendon and the tibial condyle.

29

Two bursae lie superficially to the collateral ligaments: one between the fibular collateral ligament and the overlying biceps tendon and the other between the tibial collateral ligament and the three overlying tendons of the pes anserinus (the sartorius, gracilis, and semitendinosus). One bursa exists between the superficial and the deep parts of the tibial collateral ligaments. Irritation, inflammation, and infection of these bursae must be considered in the differential diagnosis of knee pain (see Chapter 6).

A pain in the posterior knee frequently can present itself; its causation and exact area is not always clear. This is the so-called Baker's cyst. Numerous posterior bursal inflammations are so

FIGURE 26. Standing balance. With nonfunctioning quadriceps, stance is possible by ligamentous support (the posterior popliteal capsule and anterior (hip joint capsule) Y ligament of Bigelow) and by gastrocnemius action. In the weight-bearing position the gastrocnemius can be considered to originate from the calcaneus and insert the upper tibia and distal femur, thus extending the knee.

FIGURE 27. Bursae about the knee. Bursae noted above: *Suprapatellar,* also termed the quadriceps femoral bursa, may communicate with the knee capsule; *Prepatellar,* between the skin and patella; *Infrapatellar* (superficial), between the skin and infrapatellar ligament; *Deep Infrapatellar,* between infrapatellar ligament and tibia; and bursae between the lateral head of the gastrocnemius and the joint capsule, the fibular collateral ligament and the biceps or popliteal tendon, and the popliteal tendon and the lateral femoral condyle. X indicates possible communication with the joint capsule.

termed. These may include bursitis between the medial head of the gastrocnemius and the semimembranosus tendon, which may communicate with the capsule space; a synovial cyst of the semitendinosus tendon; or more important may resemble a cyst and instead be an aneurysm of the popliteal artery, an A-V fistula, or a soft tissue tumor. Proper diagnosis frequently is followed by exploratory or curative surgery.

BIBLIOGRAPHY

Basmajian, J. V.: Grant's Method of Anatomy. Williams & Wilkins, Baltimore, 1971.
Basmajian, J. V., and Lovejoy, J. F.: Function of the popliteus muscle in man. J. Bone Joint Surg. [Am] 53:557, 1971.
Brantigan, O. C., and Voshell, A. F.: Tibial collateral ligament: Its function, its bursae, and its relation to the medial meniscus. J. Bone Joint Surg. 25:1, 1943.
De Palma, A. F.: Diseases of the Knee: Management and Surgery. J. B. Lippincott Company, Philadelphia, 1954.
Helfet, A. J.: Mechanism of derangements of the medial semilunar cartilage and their management. J. Bone Joint Surg. [Br] 41:319, 1959.
Helfet, A. J.: Function of cruciate ligaments of knee-joint. Lancet 1:665, 1948.
Last, R. J.: Some anatomical details of the knee joint. J. Bone Joint Surg. [Br] 30:683, 1948.
Lieb, F. J., and Perry, J.: Quadriceps function. An electromyographic study under isometric conditions. J. Bone Joint Surg. [Am] 53:749, 1971.
Marshal, J. L., Girgis, F. G., and Zelko, R. R.: The biceps femoris tendon and its functional significance. J. Bone Joint Surg. [Am] 54:1444, 1972.
Ricklin, P., Ruttmann, A., and Del Buono, M.S.: Meniscus Lesions: Practical Problems of Clinical Diagnosis, Arthrography, and Therapy. Grune & Stratton, Inc., New York, 1971.
Slocum, D. B., and Larson, R. L.: Rotatory instability of the knee. J. Bone Joint Surg. [Am] 50:211, 1968.
Thorek, S. L.: Orthopaedics: Principles and Their Application, ed. 2. J. B. Lippincott Company, Philadelphia, 1967.

CHAPTER 2

Functional Anatomy

Knee flexion or extension is accompanied by a gliding motion of the tibia upon the femur with simultaneous rotation. There is external rotation of the tibia upon the femur during knee extension and internal rotation during flexion. The first 20° of flexion causes a rocking motion. After 20°, further flexion is composed of a gliding motion (Fig. 28).

After 20° of flexion the ligaments become relaxed and permit both gliding and axial rotation. Most rotation occurs during the final phase of full flexion and during the last 30° to 40° of extension. Some rotation, however, occurs throughout the entire flexion and extension action. At 90° of flexion 40° of rotation is possible. In full extension *no* axial rotation is possible and *no* significant lateral or medial adduction-abduction of the tibia upon the femur is possible (Fig. 29).

Rotation of the tibia upon the femur during flexion-extension is passive because of the anatomical configuration of the articular surfaces. The muscles acting upon the joint all have a rotatory torque action but this is secondary. During flexion-extension the tibia follows the configuration of the medial condyle of the femur which is longer than the lateral condyle (Fig. 30).

As the femur glides upon the tibia it stops when the surface contour of the lateral condyle has been traversed but continues to move along the longer and more curved medial condyle, which curves in a lateral direction. During extension the tibia rotates upon the femur a distance equal to half the width of the patella (Fig. 31). The knee extensors (quadriceps) run medially and thus help rotate the tibia during extension (see Fig. 14).

Flexion, from the fully extended position, begins with simultaneous internal rotation (tibia upon the femur) by contraction of the popliteus muscle. Further active flexion results from ham-

33

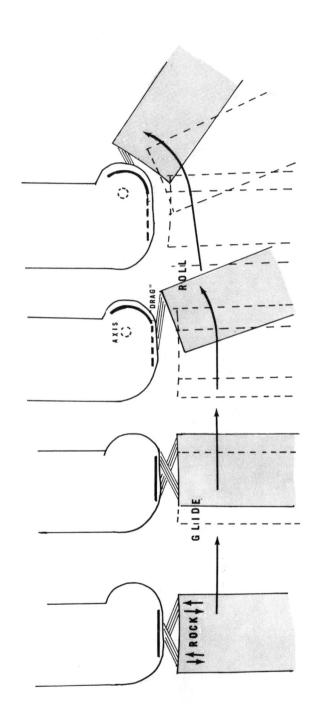

FIGURE 28. Mechanism of knee flexion. The movement of first 20° of flexion is essentially that of rocking. After 20° the femur glides upon the tibia until the rounded posterior condyles roll upon the tibial plateau. The posterior cruciate ligament relaxes during initiation of flexion, then acts as a drag to assist further flexion.

34

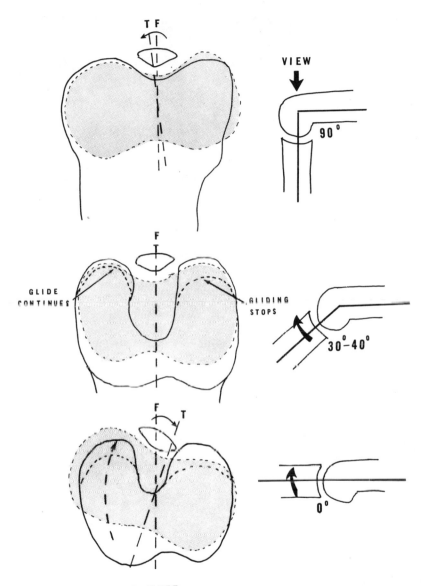

RIGHT KNEE

FIGURE 29.   Functional evaluation of knee flexion-extension. With knee flexed to 90°, 40° of rotation is possible. Active flexion has simultaneous internal rotation. *Below,* In full extension the tibia is externally rotated upon the femur.

35

FIGURE 30.   Passive mechanism of flexion-extension. *1*, The lateral condyle of the femur, L_A-L_P, is shorter than the medial condyle, M_A-M_P, thus the femur travels further on the medial surface as the quadriceps muscle continues to contract when the lateral motion ceases. Motion continues about half an inch and the femur continues to move upon the tibia, causing the tibia to rotate externally (outward). *2*, The knee is stable in full extension. The flat anterior surface of the femoral condyles fit into the tibial condyles and the ligaments are taut. The tibial intercondylar eminences prevent lateral gliding.

36

string contraction. The capsular ligaments, which are taut during full extension, relax as flexion begins. The femur glides forward upon the tibia (see Fig. 30), placing the smaller rounded posterior surface of the femoral condyles upon the tibial plateau.

The posterior cruciate ligament becomes taut (see Fig. 8) and acts as a drag to any further forward gliding. An axis now exists around which the tibia rotates upon the femur.

In flexion and extension the menisci, fixed to the tibia, move with it upon the femur. In rotation, with the knee flexed, the menisci move with the femur upon the tibia. If the femoral-meniscotibial spaces are considered to be joint spaces the upper femoral-meniscal joint moves during flexion-extension and rotation occurs at the lower meniscotibial joint (see Fig. 12).

The menisci have firm ligamentous attachments. The medial meniscus is attached at both horns and along its entire outer circumferential border. The lateral meniscus is attached at both horns but the remainder of its lateral (outer) margin is free.

The cruciate ligaments crisscross. The anterior cruciate is

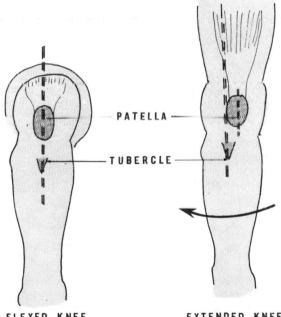

PATELLA

TUBERCLE

FLEXED KNEE   EXTENDED KNEE

FIGURE 31. Surface manifestation of tibial rotation. When the flexed knee is viewed from the front, the patella lies directly over the tibial tubercle. With the knee fully extended the tubercle is lateral to the patella, indicating external rotation during knee extension.

37

taut during extension and unwinds and relaxes during flexion. The collateral ligaments, also taut during extension, relax during flexion — the lateral more than the medial (Fig. 32). As ligamentous relaxation occurs during flexion some axial rotation is permitted and the axis of rotation moves posteriorly (Fig. 33).

The external rotation of the tibia upon the femur during the last 20° of extension is termed the "screw home" mechanism and, as stated, is due to condylar configuration, muscle torque action, and ligamentous guidance.

When the knee extends because of contraction of the quadriceps, the patella is forcefully pulled upward. The infrapatellar

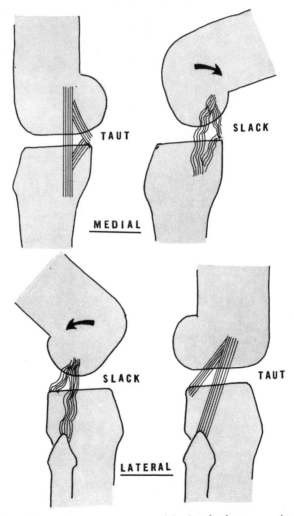

FIGURE 32. Ligamentous tautness and laxity during extension-flexion.

38

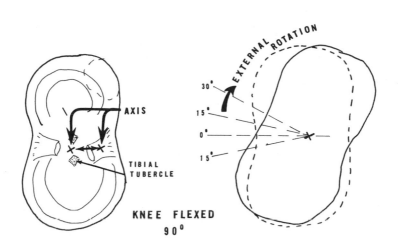

FIGURE 33. Axis of gliding and rotation. As the femur glides upon the tibia the axis of axial rotation shifts. The degree of axial rotation varies according to the degree of flexion. None (0°) is possible at full extension or complete hyperflexion. Gradual rotation is possible until 90° of flexion is reached: 30° to 40° of rotation is possible at this point of flexion with more external rotation than internal.

fat pad and the alar ligaments connected to the joint capsule are also pulled anterior and upwards, thus preventing their being impinged between the opposing condyles. The three facets on the dorsal surface of the patella simultaneously alternate their contact with the femoral patellar surface. From flexion to extension the contact goes from superior facet to middle to inferior.

Muscular action in extension is essentially that of the quadriceps femoris group. The rectus femoris alone cannot fully extend the leg; the vasti, especially the vastus medialis, perform this function. The patella mechanically increases the efficacy of the extensor mechanism by improving leverage.

The ligaments aid in knee extension. When the tibia is fixed from the foot being weight bearing, the anterior cruciate acts as a guide wire as the knee approaches full extension. When the femur is fixed the anterior cruciate controls lateral rotation of the tibia. As the knee moves from flexion to extension the motion of the lateral condyle is stopped at 160° by the anterior cruciate and the lateral collateral ligament. Continued quadriceps contraction causes the medial condyle to move the additional 20° (to full 180°) and externally rotates the tibia upon the femur.

39

CHAPTER 3

Meniscus Injuries

Many factors are involved in injury of a meniscus. The exact pathomechanics is not always clearly ascertained by a careful history nor an exacting examination.

The medial meniscus sustains injury more often than does the lateral in a ratio of 3:1. Smillie places the injury in athletes as 3:1 but other authors place it as high as 8:1. Injury of the medial over the lateral meniscus in miners has been placed as high as 20:1. The difference in ratios is correlated to the particular movements and positions of these varied professions and activities.

In studying mechanical etiological factors it is considered that damage to the meniscus occurs from compressive forces, traction forces, or a combination of both. Injury results from weight bearing upon the knee combined with faulty, forceful, or excessive motion either in flexion-rotation or extension-rotation. The combination of weight bearing *with* rotatory stress during flexion or extension as a cause of meniscus injury appears to be well accepted.

In previous chapters it was stated that the fully extended knee with normal musculature and ligamentous structure is stable. No significant lateral nor rotatory motion is possible unless an overwhelming force tears the ligaments or causes a fracture or dislocation.

During normal motion, flexion is accompanied by internal rotation of the tibia upon the femur — extension accompanied by external rotation. The ligaments alternately slacken or become taut; the menisci move appropriately forward in extension and backward in flexion.

The medial meniscus, being firmly attached around its entire periphery, moves less than the lateral meniscus, which is more centrally attached. By virtue of greater mobility the lateral meniscus sustains less injury.

During flexion and extension of the knee the menisci move anteriorly and posteriorly respectively. With maximum flexion the posterior portions of the menisci are compressed between the posterior aspects of the tibial and femoral condyles. Internal rotation of the femur upon the tibia in this flexed position will force the posterior segment of the medial meniscus towards the center of the joint space. Sudden extension of the knee can trap its posterior horn and create traction upon the entrapped meniscus. A longitudinal tear results in the meniscus (Fig. 34). The more mobile lateral meniscus can escape this entrapment and subsequent longitudinal tear.

External rotation of the femur upon the tibia in the bent knee position displaces the posterior horn of the lateral meniscus towards the center of the joint. Extension of the knee in this position of rotation, contrary to the resultant injury to the medial meniscus, does not cause a longitudinal tear but rather straightens (elongates) the lateral meniscus, placing strain upon the inner concave margin of the meniscus and tearing it transversely or obliquely (see Fig. 34).

Tearing of the meniscus with the knee fully extended is rare unless the tearing is a part of an extensive injury that disrupts the cruciate or collateral ligaments with or without condylar fracture.

The causative mechanism, therefore, must be considered to be flexion and extension of the knee, combined with forceful internal or external rotation that occurs when the tibia is fixed to the ground in a weight-bearing posture; thus the leg cannot avoid or minimize the torsion stress. From the crouched position with knees fully or even hyperflexed the femur must internally rotate upon the tibia during re-extension to the erect posture.

Another theory postulated to explain the mechanism of meniscus tear is that, combined with flexion and external rotation, a *forced valgus* of the knee (Fig. 35) occurs in which the medial joint space is opened. The opposing femoral and tibial condyle now grasp (as would a pair of pliers) the entrapped meniscus, which intrudes into the open medial joint space. The meniscus is crushed, creating a longitudinal tear and displacing the inner fragment of the posterior horn into the joint. This theory is made more plausible because the deeper, more concave, surface of the medial tibial articular condyle allows easier access of the meniscus into this space (see Fig. 1).

41

INTERNAL — ROTATION — EXTERNAL

FORCEFUL
KNEE EXTENSION

Fig. 34. (Legend appears on facing page.)

FIGURE 34. Mechanism of meniscus tear. *1*, With the knee fully flexed and the femur *internally* rotated the medial menuscus is displaced posteriorly and the posterior horn, *X*, moves towards the center. Forceful extension of the knee causes a longitudinal tearing because of the meniscus capsular attachment and/or tear of the posterior attachment. *2*, With the knee fully flexed and the femur *externally* rotated the lateral meniscus is moved posteriorly and its posterior horn towards the center of the joint. Forceful knee extension *elongates* the meniscus, causing radial tearing on the medial (inner) margin of the meniscus.

A complete longitudinal tear is rare in an initial injury to a normal meniscus but may be extended by repeated injuries. This sequence is questioned by some authorities. The fact that the undersurface of the meniscus reveals the early site of damage is probably explained by the fact that the cartilage moves with the femur, thus causing irritation by the tibial surface.

Undoubtedly there are other factors, such as constitutional inadequacy, ligamentous laxity, muscular inadequacy, faulty stressful work habits, obesity, excessive knee valgus or varus that place unequal stress upon knee structures, and violent sports, that contribute to meniscus tear and degenerative changes. Most of these ideas are conjectural but plausible. Frequently unrecognized meniscus injury occurs concurrently with tibial plateau fractures when the presence of the fracture obscures the meniscus lesion.

NORMAL   VALGUS FLEXED   EXTENSION

FIGURE 35. Valgus theory of meniscus tear. The combination of knee flexion with forced valgus, which opens the medial aspect of the knee joint, plus the deeper, more concave, tibial condyle, forces the meniscus towards the center of the joint. Re-extension pinches the entrapped meniscus between the opposing condyles.

The initial tear of the medial meniscus occurs most often in the posterior pole. If the longitudinal tear occurs exclusively in the posterior third of the meniscus, by virtue of its inherent elasticity the meniscus springs back into its normal position.

If the tear is extensive and extends anteriorly past the collateral ligament it bunches up between the two condyles and causes a locking of the knee joint.

In an extensive tear the entire inner fragment may be displaced to the center of the joint, in which case no locking results because the central fragment resides in the intercondylar fossa (Fig. 36).

Symptoms are *not* caused by the cartilage tear per se but by stretching or tearing its peripheral attachments and the acute synovial reaction within the joint space. The severity of the meniscus injury does *not* necessarily relate to the severity of the pain.

Synovial effusion invariably accompanies meniscus tears and results from injury to the synovium, the capsule, or ligaments. It is not due to tearing of the fibrocartilaginous meniscus. It must be remembered that knee injuries other than meniscus tears can cause effusion and must be considered in the differential diagnosis of a swollen knee. A large effusion may give the feeling of tightness with no pain. Hemarthrosis almost always gives severe pain.

Tears in the substance of the avascular portion of the cartilage *do not* heal. Tears in the peripheral zones heal by invasion of fibrous tissue. The meniscus removed by meniscectomy is replaced by dense collagen tissue from the remaining portion of the meniscus.

DIAGNOSTIC SIGNS AND SYMPTOMS

The history given by the patient or by an observer at the time of injury is often that of a twisting, turning movement of the leg with the foot firmly fixed to the ground (as in an athlete's quick turn in a running event), a direct blow to the turned flexed extremity, or coming to an erect posture from a full crouched position. The exact history may not be evident to the patient who attributes the injury to the fall that follows the meniscus knee injury.

Pain is usually severe and sudden as if "something tore within the knee." Pain from an acute tear of the meniscus usually causes immediate cessation of activity whereas a ligamentous sprain permits continuation albeit with discomfort. Swelling occurs within hours and occasionally the knee locks immediately but the locking may be momentary and suddenly, spontaneously, reduced.

Effusion is usually present following the initial injury. Without effusion, an extra-articular lesion must be suspected. Lesions of the lateral meniscus cause less effusion than the medial cartilage because of having less peripheral capsular attachment. Immediate massive bloody effusion implies severe capsular, ligamentous and/or bony injury.

Tenderness may be elicited along the entire joint line, which probably indicates tearing of the peripheral attachment of the meniscus. Tenderness is present mostly in the posterior area of the knee joint. Rarely is there tenderness anteriorly as tearing usually does not occur there. In meniscus tear tenderness may be in the region of the medial collateral ligament but tear of the ligament, with or without associated meniscus injury, causes tenderness *above* the joint line.

Locking is rare in an initial injury as the tear is usually in the posterior third of the meniscus with no displacement or bunching of the cartilage (see Fig. 36). In more severe initial tears or repeated tearing injuries, which extend anteriorly to or past the coronal plane of the joint, locking can result, thus preventing *full extension of the knee.* True locking is usually sudden and unlocking may be equally sudden. Gradual locking may be the result of effusion hemorrhage within the infrapatellar fat pad or from an unrecognized loose body within the joint. Not all meniscus injuries give a history of locking; in fact, 50 percent of these injuries have never locked.

Buckling, giving away of the knee, noted by the patient during the act of walking, often on irregular terrain, may indicate a tear of the posterior segment of the meniscus.

Clicking, audible to the patient or examiner, is considered to be caused by the femoral condyle riding over an articular irregularity. It must be differentiated from the grating noted in an osteoarthritic knee, in chondromalacia patellae, or when the hamstring tendon snaps over the femoral condyle.

Atrophy of the quadriceps occurs rapidly after a meniscus injury and is particularly evident in the vastus medialis. Measurable atrophy may be noted within days and certainly within two weeks following the injury.

45

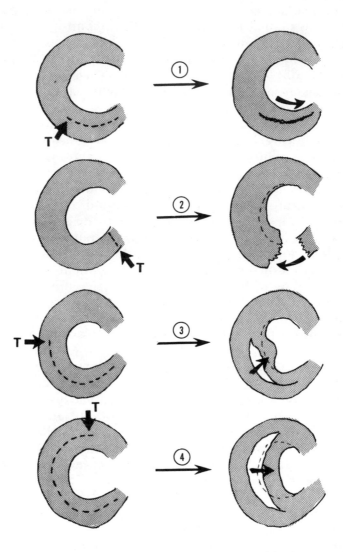

FIGURE 36.   Types of meniscus tears. *1*, With a tear within the posterior third of the meniscus, the elasticity of the cartilage springs the meniscus back into its normal position. *2*, Posterior tear, *T*, of the horn's attachment causes the anterior portion to bunch, and locking results. *3*, A tear, *T*, halfway to the collateral ligament causes a bunching of the middle portion of the meniscus with similar symptoms to *2*. *4*, If the tear, *T*, is complete (entire length of the meniscus) the central portion of the meniscus moves towards the center of the joint. This is called a bucket handle tear. No locking occurs because the central fragment is in the intercondylar fossa.

So-called *meniscus signs* are numerous and vary depending upon the author being studied. Unfortunately these signs employ the proper name of the physician who initially described that particular test. A physiological basis for any test makes the examination and its interpretation more meaningful.

McMurray sign. This is a time-honored test in which the patient in the recumbent position has the knee flexed until the heel touches (or approaches) the buttocks (Fig. 37). To test the medial meniscus the leg is externally rotated upon the femur (internally rotated to test the lateral meniscus). The leg is gradually extended with rotation forcefully maintained. The test is valid only during extension from 90° of flexion and does not diagnose tears in the anterior one third of the meniscus.

Apley Test. This test aims at differentiating a meniscus lesion from capsular or ligamentous injury. With the patient prone the knee is flexed to 90° and the leg is rotated with simultaneous upward traction. Pain with this maneuver implies capsular or ligamentous injury. Rotation of the bent knee with downward pressure causing pain or "clicking" indicates a meniscus lesion (see Fig. 37).

Steinmann's Tenderness Displacement Sign. Tenderness is displaced posteriorly as the knee is flexed, anteriorly as the knee is extended (Fig. 38). The site of tenderness does not shift in degenerative osteoarthrosis of the knee.

Hyperflexion Meniscus Test. With the patient prone and hyperflexing the knee (Fig. 39), with the lower leg in internal or external rotation, may cause the cartilage to slip forward and cause a painful click as the opposing condyles compress the fragment.

There are many other tests for meniscus lesions but all are founded on the same mechanical basis. With the understanding of the mechanics of the underlying pathology the examiner should familiarize himself with proper consistent examination and become proficient in a careful technique in order to assure a meaningful examination.

Arthrography

The diagnostic procedure of injecting dye into the joint and thus outlining all intra-articular tissues is gaining more advocates and is becoming a gratifying procedure. Full detail and dis-

47

FIG. 37. (Legend appears on facing page.)

48

FIGURE 37. Meniscus signs (examination). *1, 2, 3, McMurray test.* The patient is supine with knee fully flexed, heel touching the buttocks at the start. The leg is internally rotated for lateral meniscus testing or externally rotated for medial meniscus testing. Then the knee is fully extended. A painful click occurs if there is a meniscus lesion. The test is more meaningful in the first phase of knee extension. Full extension limitation does not indicate an anterior meniscus lesion. *4, 5, Apley test.* The patient is prone. Leg is internally or externally rotated with simultaneous traction. Pain indicates a capsular or ligamentous lesion. Rotation with downward pressure that causes pain indicates meniscus lesion.

cussion of the numerous interpretations made possible by this test is beyond the scope of this monograph but certain principals are indicated.

Many pitfalls, which may lead to faulty diagnosis or unwarranted negative conclusions, exist in the interpretation of an arthrogram. Therefore the test should be performed and interpreted by an experienced diagnostic radiologist or trained orthopedist.

Before arthrography is performed the joint should be evacuated as completely as possible of all intra-articular fluid. Air then is injected into the joint to distend the capsule and create a fluoroscopic contrast. Twenty to forty cubic centimeters of air can safely and painlessly be injected, but the exact amount should be restricted to that amount which causes no painful distension yet good visible contrast in the joint. After the air is injected, 3 to 4 cc. of liquid contrast medium is injected through the same needle. The needle is then withdrawn.

The patient is instructed to fully move his knee after the injection. He should *not* put weight on that leg. However, he may stand on the other leg and allow the injected knee to be dependent. These numerous movements insure the dyecoating of all intra-articular tissues. Not only the menisci and intra-articular ligaments may be visualized but also the bursae that connect with the joint space. Several examples will be graphically illustrated to explain the principals of arthrography (Figs. 40 and 41). Currently much literature on the subject is being published.

TREATMENT

Tears into the meniscus that do not extend into the peripheral vascular portion of the fibrocartilage do not heal. Those that do extend into the vascular zone heal if there is reduction of the

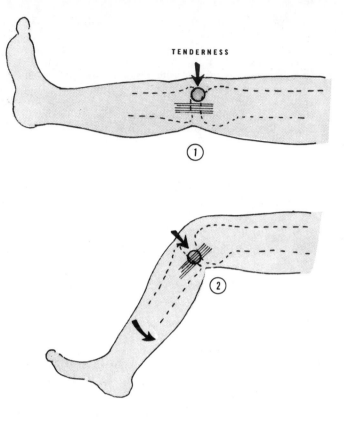

FIGURE 38. Meniscus sign: tenderness displacement test. *1*, With the extended knee the tenderness over the medial meniscus occurs anteriorly. *2*, As the knee is flexed the tenderness migrates posteriorly towards the medial collateral ligament.

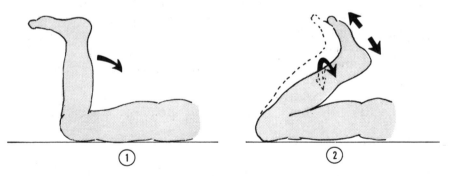

FIGURE 39. Hyperflexion meniscus test. With the patient prone the knee is flexed to 90°. Then, with internal or external rotation of the leg upon the femur, the knee is *hyperflexed*. Painful clicking may indicate a posterior meniscus tear. Doing this maneuver may cause the knee to lock from movement of the fragment into the joint.

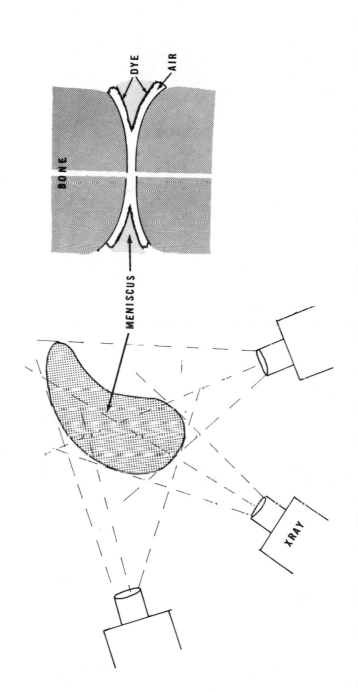

FIGURE 40. Arthrography. The knee, and thus the meniscus, is rotated before the X ray so that both poles and the entire meniscus are visualized. *Left*, The lateral and medial aspects of the joint are visualized separately; *Right*, The air creates contrast and the dye coats all intra-articular tissues.

51

displaced meniscus and the knee is immobilized for at least three weeks. In an obvious tear, i.e., one with incomplete extension indicating medial displacement, conservative treatment must be viewed as temporary, permitting merely painfree return of function, but futile if disability and pain recur.

The decision regarding surgery varies with the surgeon's experience and no hard-fast rules are applicable. In general, however, the locking knee with recurrences should have arthrotomy.

Reduction

The locked knee must be reduced within twenty-four hours. After this time the effusion causes a loss of elasticity of the meniscus and prevents its springing back into normal position. This reduction manipulation (Fig. 42) usually does not require an anesthetic. The technique is (1) apply longitudinal traction with simultaneous rotation in both directions and lateral motion (valgus and varus stress) with leg principally in *valgus* position; (2) full flexion of the knee with forceful internal rotation if the medial meniscus is being treated (external rotation if the lateral

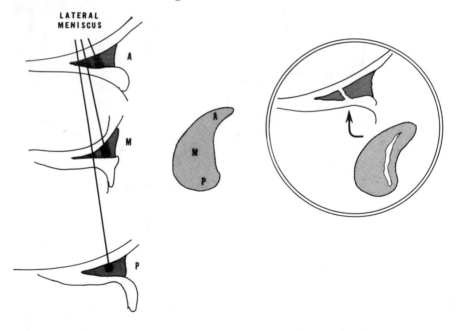

FIGURE 41.   Arthrograms. *Center,* Normal lateral menisci: *A,* Anterior horn; *M,* Middle horn; *P,* Posterior horn. *Left,* What is seen on lateral x-ray pictures; *Right,* An arthrogram taken of a torn meniscus.

meniscus); and (3) forceful kicking (extension) by the patient. Achieving full free range of motion indicates a reduction (unlocking). The range must be compared with the other leg to ascertain full extension as compared to normal.

Repeated unsuccessful manipulations may cause extension of the tear anteriorly or centrally into the joint space (see Fig. 36). If there is persistence of a displaced fragment the last few degrees of extension are both actively and passively prevented. *Forceful attempts must be avoided* and weight bearing should not be permittted.

FIGURE 42.   Manipulation of "locked knee." The purpose of manipulation to unlock the meniscus is to relieve pain and prevent further damage to the meniscus. *A*, In lateral meniscus the knee is fully flexed and some pressure is exerted to cause varus of the leg (*M*, medial pressure; *L*, lateral pressure). *D*, The leg is externally rotated. Then the surgeon suddenly (but not forcefully) extends the leg *A* to *B*. For lesions of the medial meniscus the opposite motion (internal rotation varus) is used.

53

Conservative treatment is permissible; in fact it is indicated if full extension is possible when a definite diagnosis is not possible immediately following the initial injury. A more careful examination is possible after the effusion has subsided, the quadriceps tone has returned, and function appears possible. If full range of motion is possible ambulation for testing is permitted.

If manipulation has reduced the locking a rehabilitation program of exercises (to be described later) may be started. Deep knee bends and squats are to be avoided as are sports activities.

In addition to a meniscus tear there may be tearing or severe sprain of the collateral or cruciate ligamentous structures. An evaluation of these structures must be carefully made as well as performing the meniscus signs.

In the absence of locking, two or three weeks of conservative treatment will reduce or remove the effusion and permit accurate evaluation. If there is an associated ligamentous lesion *with* a locked knee the knee must first be unlocked. The purpose of conservative treatment is to promote absorption of the effusion, restoration of the quadriceps mechanism, and immediate unlocking of the joint.

The unlocking has been described. Removal of the effusion is undertaken by initial application of ice packs for 24 to 36 hours followed by heat (whirlpool, hot moist packs, diathermy, etc.), aspiration with or without simultaneous instillation of hyaluronidase, avoidance of weight bearing (through use of crutches, wheel chair, etc.), and avoidance of compression dressings. Quadriceps function maintenance or restoration will be discussed in the postoperative section.

Surgery

Surgical technique is beyond the scope of this treatise and reference is made to the many excellent orthopedic texts and to scientific articles in orthopedic journals. Surgical failures in which the results are poor (knee instability, persistent pain and limitation, recurrent effusion, etc.) are caused by:

1. Improper or incomplete diagnosis.
2. Incompetent surgical technique.
3. Excessively prolonged conservative treatment with repeated episodes of locking or giving way.

4. Meniscus injury in a knee exhibiting severe degenerative osteoarthritic changes.
5. Removal of only *one* of the affected menisci.
6. Incomplete removal of the meniscus. (This indication is disputed in current literature.)
7. Inadequate postoperative treatment.

Postoperative Rehabilitation Program. Immediately postoperative, before the tourniquet is removed, the leg should be firmly wrapped in a compression dressing and elevated. On the second day quadriceps setting exercises should be started. These should be done for 10 to 15 minutes 3 to 4 times daily. When possible, at elective surgery or time permitting, instruction in these exercises *preoperatively* facilitates their being understood and properly done postoperatively. From the third day, the patient should progress from isometric exercises to straight leg raising, using the weight of the leg for resistance. Then he should progress to increased resistance as tolerated with encouragement and supervision so that failure to progress is not permitted. Excessive pain and/or effusion should cause review of the program. Normal use is usual within ten weeks.

Quadriceps Exercises

Exercise to strengthen the quadriceps mechanism is of sufficient importance to devote space to a full discussion and detail. The question is that of power versus endurance: which to stress? How is it attainable? Which is important?

Power building exercises do not develop endurance, but power is essential and should be developed first. The rate of development of muscle volume (mass), and thus power, is proportional to the resistance imposed upon the muscle. Heavy resistance exercise with low repetition creates power; low resistance with high repetition creates endurance. The greater the stretch (elongation) of the muscle the greater the contractile power; thus in the stretched position fewer fibers are used than when contraction is in the shortened position. Maximum tension occurs at lengths 10 percent longer than the resting length.

Strength increase occurs by the recruitment of additional motor units rather than by more rapid firing of the contracting units. Therefore strength increase depends upon (1) greater voluntary effort, (2) integrity of the central nervous system, and (3) better synaptic and endplate function. Only the first is directly influenced by patient effort.

Progressive resistive exercises are essentially rhythmic *dynamic* exercises. They use maximum resistance (load) and are gradually upgraded as strength improves. A prescribed increase in daily series moves the muscle through its full range of motion and insures proper positioning so that only the prime movers of that joint are treated.

Static (muscle setting) exercises have their greatest value where joint motion needs to be avoided or is not possible. *Isokinetic exercises* attempt a combination of isotonic (kinetic) and isometric (static) exercises in which speed of motion is kept constant by equipment and maximum tension is applied and maintained through the entire cycle. This type of exercise is still in the experimental stage and cannot be fully evaluated.

The types of exercises and their exact application vary with the stage of the recovery or postoperative state. Early in postsprain condition, postoperatively when joint motion is not desired, or with leg in a pressure dressing or cast when joint motion is not wanted, *isometric setting exercises* are advisable. The term "isometric" is a misnomer, implying no movement when there is motion of the muscle and the patella. Only joint motion is excluded.

In chondromalacia patellae, where quadriceps exercises must be performed with minimal or no patellar movement, the quadriceps should be slowly and fully contracted before maximum contraction (setting) is attempted. Straight leg raising against resistance is effective here. With the leg fully extended have the patient contract the quadriceps muscle to its maximum with the greatest effort tolerated. Motion is judged by observing the upward motion of the patella, bulging or firming of the quadriceps muscle. The contraction should be sustained for a count to 3 or 5, then relaxed. This exercise is performed 15 to 30 times every hour of the waking day with attempt at increasing the effort of contraction.

Straight leg raising without resistance is begun when setting has been mastered and strength, as observed by muscle bulk, appears to be returning. Straight leg raising should be done hourly with sustained elevation at 45° and an intermittent rest period. Recent studies (Ladley) show that this straight leg raising is a less effective progressive form of exercise than resisted extension with knee slightly flexed over a supporting block (Fig. 43).

Straight leg raising against elastic resistance or sand bags of graded weights are then instituted. Postoperative resistance exercises are not started for 3 to 4 weeks after surgery but setting

56

exercises should be started the first postoperative day, with straight leg raising begun as soon as tolerated by the patient even though the leg may be in a pressure dressing or cast.

Progress to resistance exercises of a kinetic type (with range of motion of the joint) is based on certain concepts and approved methods. Resistance is applied either manually by a physical therapist or trained relative or with mechanical equipment. Several concepts need clarification before the progressive resistive program is detailed. As stated previously, quadriceps setting with knee fully extended is not considered to be the most effective method. By placing a small, well-padded block of less than 3 inches in thickness under the knee, flexing the knee very slightly, exercise seems more effective as ascertained by electromyographic surface electrodes (see Fig. 43). The position or action of the foot, simultaneous plantar flexion, dorsiflexion, inversion, or eversion during quadriceps exercises have been

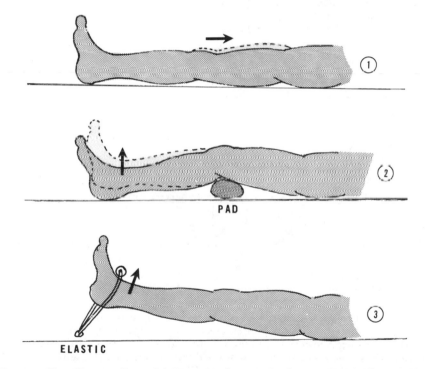

FIGURE 43. Types of quadriceps exercises. *1*, Setting or isometric exercises with knee fully extended. Joint does not move but muscle shortens: patella moves up. *2*, Isometric (kinetic) exercise. With a 3-inch thick pad under the knee the quadriceps contracts. The joint range of motion is minimal and quadriceps function is enhanced over *1*. *3*, Increase in exercise with an elastic strap to resist straight leg raising.

questioned. It appears that concurrent ankle dorsiflexion enhances the quadriceps efficiency.

The essence of progressive resistance exercise (P.R.E.) (Delorme) is the determination of the maximum resistance that the patient can overcome to full extension for one contraction (called 1 R.M.) and the determination of the weight that can be lifted to full extension for ten repeated efforts (10 R.M.). As the

FIGURE 44. Progressive resistive exercises. *Above,* The standard technique of P.R.E. with a weighted boot. Full extension is attempted, *A,* and briefly sustained. *B,* The leg is lowered until the weight and foot are supported to prevent ligamentous stress. *B* causes exercise toward extension from the semi-extended position, where the vastus medialis is most effective, rather than from *C,* where resistance against the quadriceps is minimal as the weight pulls vertically along the tibial shaft. In the *C* position there is a greater chance of stress upon the ligaments of the knee from the weighted dependent leg. *Below,* Resistance with pulleys and weight places maximum resistance in the first 45° of extension, *Y,* and decreases as the leg extends, thus placing none (0°) at full extension, *X.*

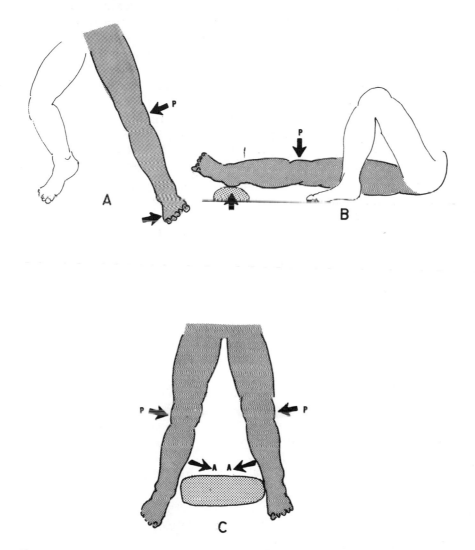

FIGURE 45. Exercises to stress ligaments of the knee. Both medial and lateral collateral ligaments are stretched daily as part of the exercise program on the assumption that gentle but firm and repeated stress upon the ligaments increases their resilience. *A* and *B,* Indicate how the patient stretches manually the medial ligament. *C,* With the use of a firm pillow both active, *A,* and passive, *P,* exercises stretch and stress the ligaments. Exercises weighted against gravity also stress and strengthen ligaments.

program progresses the weight of 10 R.M. attached to the foot and allowed to rest on a support between lifts is raised to full knee extension and then lowered slowly back to the support for a period of rest for 1 to 2 minutes. It is again lifted. At the extreme of full extension, maximum effort is exerted to recruit all motor units and the leg is held extended for the count of three. The exercise period lasts 30 to 45 minutes and is done three times a day. Heat and massage is beneficial following each series.

The resistance is gradually increased and the repetitions decreased. The 10 R.M.s are determined every week, with increase in increments of $\frac{1}{4}$ to $\frac{1}{2}$ lb. as tolerated up to 1 lb. Gradually a weight that permits merely one full excursion is reached; this is 1 R.M. and requires maximum effort. This lift is done three times daily and followed by rest, heat, and massage if desired. This weight is also gradually increased. A weight of 30 to 35 lb. can be reached in most adults; more in athletes. Normal power is usually reached in 3 to 6 weeks.

Power having been or being reached, it is now desirable that endurance exercises be initiated. These include bicycling, stair climbing and descending, jumping jacks, shallow knee bends (*never to exceed 50 percent of a full squat*), and jogging.

The use of a weight applied to the foot-ankle rather than the use of a pulley needs clarification (Fig. 44). Resistance from the weighted boot is maximum in the most effective range of extension: the last 45°. By lowering the boot to the support after each lift no ligamentous strain or stretch to the ligaments occurs. The resistance from the pulley is maximum at the beginning of knee extension when the knee is flexed 90° but decreases as the knee extends.

Exercises are also considered to be effective in increasing the tensile strength of ligaments. As the quadriceps' power returns, gentle stress upon the ligaments should be incorporated in the exercise program (Fig. 45). *Gentle* manual pressure upon the leg in a valgus or varus direction is taught the patient in addition to side-lying abduction-adduction exercises against a weighted boot. Prone progressive resistance exercises to the hamstrings are beneficial.

BIBLIOGRAPHY

Delorme, T. L.: Restoration of muscle power by heavy resistance exercises. J. Bone Joint Surg. 27:645, 1945.

Dickinson, A. L.: Resistance exercises for development of strength of muscles that extend leg at knee: A comparative study of three methods. Ph.D. Dissertation. State University of Iowa, Iowa City, 1962.

King, D.: The healing of semilunar cartilage. J. Bone Joint Surg. 18:333, 1936.

Klein, K. K.: A continuation study of specific progressive resistance exercises for increasing medial lateral collateral ligamentous stability. J. Assoc. Physical Mental Rehab. 19:162, 1965.

Ladley, G.: An investigation into the effectiveness of various forms of quadriceps exercises. Physiotherapy. 57:356, 1971.

Schaer, H.: Der Meniscusschaden. G. Thieme, Leipsig, 1938.

CHAPTER 4

Ligamentous Injuries

Ligaments are fibrous collagen tissues properly employed about a joint to prevent abnormal or excessive motion of that joint. Excessive joint motion that causes injury to the ligaments constitutes a *sprain*. Sprains may vary from complete tear of the ligament, with or without avulsion of the fragment of bone to which it is attached, to merely minor tearing of a few fibers without loss of integrity of the ligament. Tears within a ligament may be longitudinal, transverse, or oblique, causing elongation of the remaining ligamentous fibers. *Strain* semantically may be considered to be the physical force imposed upon the ligamentous tissues possibly exceeding normal stress but not causing deformation or damage to the tissues. Physiological recovery is expected.

The knee joint sustains a sprain when a force (strain) is exerted that exceeds normal range of motion or causes an abnormal motion of the joint with tissue injury. Abnormal motion includes abduction or adduction of the extended knee, excessive rotation, hyperextension or hyperflexion, or any combination of the above. The patient may be able to describe the exact type and severity of the injury he has sustained and a witness may furnish the necessary details. Frequently neither the patient nor the witness can furnish a significant history because its significance at the time of insult is not so considered by the patient until specifically questioned.

Immediate evaluation of the injured knee is desirable because specific treatment is dependent on the severity of the injury. Was the injury considered serious by the patient? Was the patient totally disabled immediately or could he continue his activity? Was the pain mild or severe? Did the knee lock? Was effusion immediate and marked or delayed and gradual? These details indicate the severity of ligamentous injury, meniscus involvement, etc. Later, after inital injury, secondary factors of pain, effusion, guarding, concern, and faulty memory all become confusing and render the history inaccurate.

CLASSIFICATION OF DEGREE OF STRAIN

Determination of the *degree* of ligamentous injury is necessary in order to initiate proper early treatment and give a reasonable prognosis as to ultimate functional recovery, need for surgery, and/or ultimate duration of rehabilitation. Ligamentous injuries are generally classified as mild, moderate, or severe. The following classification obviously is arbitrary with much overlap and dependent upon the experience of the examiner. Basically it is:

Mild: A few fibers are torn but the integrity of the ligament is maintained and the joint remains stable.
Moderate: Fibers are torn in sufficient quantity to diminish the ligamentous function but still maintain joint stability. Some excessive joint motion is evident when compared to the other side, with some discomfort elicited.
Severe: Complete tearing of fibers with loss of integrity and evidence of joint instability.

Diagnostic Features and Treatment

Mild sprain. Pain can be elicited by stress upon the ligaments. There is tenderness, and some local swelling is noted. The joint is stable with no effusion nor locking. Certain movements that place stress on the joint may be painful.

Treatment is essentially the relief of discomfort by restricting activities and applying ice packs initially followed by heat, by compression wrapping, and through oral medication of any anti-inflammatory agent. Local injection of an anesthetic agent with or without steroids may be desirable. Oral analgesics and injection can camouflage a more severe injury and permit aggravation. Activity may be permitted if the activity is not too stressful and the patient is reliable.

Moderate sprain. Swelling is noted locally. Frequently some effusion of the joint occurs, which indicates excessive joint movement occurred at the time of injury. Pain can be elicited by stressing the joint, but normal movement may also be painful and physical limitation is self imposed. Locking may occur if there is concurrent meniscus injury or moderate joint effusion or

63

hemarthrosis. Instability can be ascertained if the involved joint is carefully compared with the opposite joint.

Treatment consists of complete resting of the knee by bedrest or a wheelchair with leg elevated and with ice packs. Any ambulation for personal needs requires crutches and *no* weight bearing on the involved leg. Ice packs are usually of value for the first 24 to 72 hours; with cessation of pain and effusion application of heat may be substituted. Pressure wrapping is valuable with the type and manner dependent on the expertise of the person treating the injury. An example of pressure wrapping is shown in Figure 46. The joint should be aspirated if effusion is moderate or marked and should be repeated if there is recurrence. Intra-articular steroids have little to offer but are advocated by some authorities as is the instillation of hyaluronidase. Weight bearing is definitely prohibited. Ultimately an exercise program should be undertaken. Application of a cast (see Fig. 46) is advisable if there is severe pain, marked effusion, and apparent instability.

Repeated aspirations must be done when bloody fluid is retrieved. If the aspirated fluid is cloudy and yellowish, aspiration may be followed by instilling steroids.

The duration of conservative treatment is not an exact feature. Three weeks must be considered as minimal in a moderately severe ligamentous sprain. Exercises of an isometric type must be started early and gradually progress into the resistive types (see Chapter 3). Gentle flexion may be started early within the restrictive confines of the cast; then, usually within five days of the removal of the cast, gentle flexion may be continued with greater range.

Persistence or aggravation of pain and/or effusion is an in-

FIGURE 46. Method of pressure dressing and casting. The leg is held behind the thigh and the heel, *1*, to permit the tibia to hang, thus relaxing the anterior cruciate ligament. First wrap is sheet wadding (or gauze), *2*, for uniform compression. A stirrup splint made of plaster strips, *3*, is used to prevent lateral motion. A posterior mold splint, *4*, with the foot dorsiflexed is then applied, and a final wrap around of gauze or 6 inches of a thin layer of plaster is used.

dication to decrease the intensity of the treatment program, especially the exercises and weight bearing. Re-examination at this stage may alter the classification of the degree of sprain.

Severe ligamentous sprain. This implies that the ligament is torn through its substance and away from its attachment with or without avulsing a piece of bone or cartilage. Disability is severe and immediate. Joint *instability* results. Swelling, if it occurs, is immediate and usually marked. Locking may occur because of a concommitent tear in a meniscus or because of the severity of the effusion. Early examination is of utmost importance before swelling, pain, and protective spasms obscure the picture. X-ray pictures with valgus or varus stress will reveal excessive motion of the joint of an unphysiological degree.

There are cardinal factors related to ligamentous injuries of the knee that clarify the interpretation of the examination. Experimentally (Palmer) the knee, with both cruciate ligaments removed, remains laterally stable in the fully extended position; excessive rocking is possible however with the knee slightly flexed. Removal of both collateral ligaments in an otherwise intact joint maintains knee stability in *hyperextension* but permits rocking with knee in slight flexion. Tear of the posterior capsule does not materially influence lateral stability. These findings imply that instability in the *hyperextended* knee position indicates damage to the cruciate ligaments and that lateral instability with the *knee flexed* indicates damage to the tibial collateral ligaments (Fig. 47).

Mere tear of the tibial collateral ligament does not cause joint lateral mobility in full extension and *no* drawer sign. (With knee flexed to 90° and foot flexed by examiner, a *positive drawer sign* implies excessive motion of the tibia upon the femur on a horizontal anteroposterior motion as compared to the other (normal) side (Fig. 48). Tear of anterior cruciate only causes *no* lateral instability but permits an increased drawer effect and allows greater knee hyperextension. Tear of the anterior cruciate ligament *and* the tibial collateral ligament allows lateral instability that increases as the knee is flexed and allows a positive drawer sign. Lateral motion of 10° to 15° with knee fully extended is possible.

A knee injury in which external rotation occurs to the already flexed knee initiates a sequence of injury: (1) initial tearing of the deep medial ligament (capsule), (2) tearing of the tibial collateral ligament, and (3) tearing of the anterior cruciate ligament (Fig. 49).

In a severe injury a bloody effusion indicates damage to internal structures of the knee as well as to the ligaments. Tearing of the tibial ligament *without* synovial damage will not cause effusion: merely local edema and ecchymosis.

In treatment of severe ligamentous injuries with resultant instability there are advocates of immediate surgery and advocates of prolonged conservative treatment. Experimentally it has been shown that ligaments in which some fibers remain and in which there is good circulation regenerate well. With poor circulation there is scar formation which is of poorer quality than ligamentous growth. Avulsion of the anterior cruciate ligament

FIGURE 47.   Severe ligamentous sprain (the unhappy triad). *1*, Lateral stress causing disruption of the medial collateral ligament, the medial meniscus, and the anterior cruciate ligament (the unhappy triad). *2*, Lateral view of a severe anterior stress causing hyperextension of the joint and disrupting both anterior and posterior cruciate ligaments and the posterior capsule. Clinically it has a positive drawer sign. *Far Right,* Arrows indicate the direction of movement by the examiner.

66

from it's femur attachment interferes with its blood supply and healing is poor; avulsion from its tibial attachment causes retraction and *no* healing.

In many cases prolonged conservative treatment will result in a stable knee but of lesser stability than the early and adequately operated knee. Even in a knee with adequate surgical repair instability frequently results, especially when there is a concomittent meniscus and/or patellar injury.

Careful consideration must be given the possibility of vascular or nerve injury when the ligamentous injuries are of significant severity to cause dislocation. The posterior popliteal artery is attached superiorly to the femur by the tendinous hiatus of the adductor magnus muscle and permits no mobility. The artery

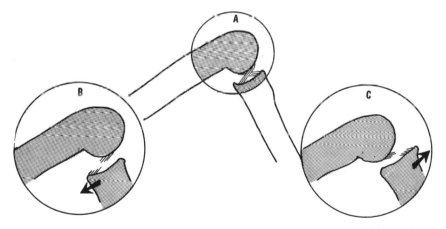

FIGURE 48. The drawer test for cruciate ligaments. *Above,* Position of the patient and the hands of the examiner in this test. The foot is fixed upon the examining table and the lower leg is horizontally moved proximally and distally. *Below, A,* The knee with intact cruciate ligaments, which move a minimal distance equal to the opposite normal leg; *B,* Tear of the posterior cruciate with the tibia moving backwards upon the femur; *C,* Movement elicited in a torn anterior cruciate. Excessive motion is possible in both directions if both cruciates are torn.

descends beneath the tendinous arch of the soleus and here it is firmly attached to the tibia. Hyperextension or shear dislocation of the knee in an anteroposterior direction can cause disruption of the artery. Lateral subluxation or severe varus injuries can damage the common peroneal nerve (Fig. 50). Conservative treatment of dislocation (Taylor et al.) has recently been claimed to give as good results as operative repair when there has been no vascular or nerve damage but merely ligamentous and capsular insult.

RUPTURE OF QUADRICEPS MECHANISM

Disruption of the quadriceps extensor mechanism may occur from direct and indirect trauma. Tear can occur in the muscle at the level of the muscle tendon junction, within the tendon, at the tendo-osseous junction of the upper or lower pole of the patella, tendon below the patella, or where the tendon attaches to the tibial tubercle.

Generally, direct trauma is caused by a forceful blow upon a contracted quadriceps muscle, usually when the knee is slightly flexed. It occurs more often in the aged or deconditioned individual. In the aged the site of avulsion is mostly a separation of the tendon from the patella. In the young the injury is usually

FIGURE 49.   Sequence of ligamentous injury. In the flexed knee (to 90°) excessive external rotation results in tearing of the capsule (deep medial ligament). The tibial collateral ligament tears under the combination of abduction stress and further rotation, and ultimately the anterior cruciate ligament tears with further stress.

from violent athletic activities and avulsion occurs mostly at the tendotubercle insertion.

The history is often that of an aged, overweight, and poorly conditioned individual who, descending stairs or jumping down, sustained a severe pain in the anterior knee area, felt or heard a snapping, and fell suddenly to the ground. Examination reveals swelling and tenderness at the site of tear. A sulcus may be

FIGURE 50. Traumatic dislocation of the knee. *A*, Lateral view of the knee with the popliteal artery adherent to the lower femur and the upper tibia; *B*, Direct injury to the femur, causing posterior luxation (shear) with arterial tear, *X*. *C*, Hyperextension injury; *D*, Common auto accident injury with flexed knee, causing the tibia to dislocate posteriorly. Here also there is blood vessel injury.

palpable. There is inability to extend the knee, unless the tear is incomplete, in which case quadriceps power is present but diminished. Type of treatment is surgical repair of the tear followed by rehabilitation exercises.

Disruption of the tendon from the tubercle may occur from direct trauma but more often it is the result of indirect injury. Clinically there is acute pain, local tenderness, probable swelling, and impaired knee extension. A gap is usually palpable and the patella, both palpably and by x-ray study, is situated higher than normal.

The indirect mechanism of injury requires some discussion. Injury to the extensor mechanism occurs when the foot is on the ground and the athlete is accelerating or decelerating his running, usually the latter. Forward motion is decelerated at foot strike of the leading leg and the knee is bent more than during the similar phase of foot-heel strike in walking. Because running is essentially a series of coordinated jumps the full body weight adds to the force of foot strikes (Fig. 51). In teenagers the epiphysis and tendons are weaker than the muscle-tendon unions, thus injury is more apt to occur at this site.

Treatment of disruption in the young may merely require immobilization in a cast for one month but, when there is sig-

A   B

FIGURE 51. Indirect injury to extensor mechanism. *A* illustrates the deceleration of the quadriceps during running at the time of leading foot strike with knee slightly bent; *B* reveals the acute stress of the quadriceps during the last phase of a jump.

nificant avulsion, surgical repair is desirable. Complications of extensor mechanism disruption by patellar dislocation or fracture will be discussed in a subsequent chapter.

MYOSITIS OSSIFICANS

This condition is a frequent complication of contusion and hematoma caused by trauma to a muscle near its insertion to the bone. The implication that myositis is inflammation within the muscle is disputed. Rather it is considered to be periosteal in origin with the muscle avulsing the periosteum and causing a periosteal hematoma that invades the overlying muscle. There may actually be a small fragment of bone and periosteum that invades the muscle and/or invasion of periosteal cells into the overlying muscle hematoma. The mass is considered pure bone directly attached to the adjacent bone or separated by a thin layer of muscle.

If rest is instituted after the trauma the blood will usually be absorbed, but continued activity, further blows, unwise massage, etc. may cause ultimate ossification. Early x-ray pictures usually are negative, thus they should be repeated within three weeks if the mass persists. Treatment is conservative to prevent further bleeding and encourage absorption. Rest is mandatory. Ice applications should be followed within several days by heat. Massage if contraindicated. Gradually instituting gentle range of motion of the knee will minimize contracture and regain quadriceps strength. Rarely is surgery indicated, even in the well-ossified masses.

BIBLIOGRAPHY

Abbott, L., Saunders, J. D., Bost, F. C., and Anderson, C.: Injuries to ligaments of the knee. J. Bone Joint Surg. 26:503, 1944.

Kennedy, J. C., and Fowler, P. J.: Medial and anterior instability of the knee. J. Bone Joint Surg. [Am] 53:7, 1971.

Meyers, M. H., and Harvey, J. P.: Traumatic dislocation of the knee joint. J. Bone Joint Surg. [Am] 53:16, 1971.

O'Donoghue, D. H.: Treatment of Injuries to Athletes. W. B. Saunders Company, Philadephia, 1962.

O'Donoghue, D. H.: Surgical treatment of fresh injuries to the major ligaments of the knee. J. Bone Joint Surg. [Am] 32:721, 1950.

Palmer, L.: On the injuries of the ligaments of the knee joints. A clinical study. Acta Chir. Scand. 81:1938.

Reynolds, F. C.: Injuries to ligaments of the knee. J. Omaha Mid-West Clin. Soc. 23:103, 1962.

Slocum, D. B., and Larson, R. L.: Pes anserinus transplantation: A surgical procedure for conrol of the rotatory instability of the knee. J. Bone Joint Surg. [Am] 50:226, 1968.

Slocum, D. B., and Larson, R. L.: Indirect injuries to the extensor mechanism of the knee in athletes. Am. J. Orthop. 6:248, 1964.

Smillie, J. S.: Injuries of the Knee Joint, ed. 2. Livingstone, Edinburgh, 1951.

Taylor, A. R., Arden, G. P., and Rainey, H. A.: Traumatic dislocation of the knee. J. Bone Joint Surg. [Br] 54:96, 1972.

CHAPTER 5

Patellar Injuries and Diseases

Injuries and diseases of the patella, which can impair this portion of the extensor mechanism of the knee, are so numerous that the subject merits separate consideration. In differentiating *injury* from *disease* it will be apparent that injury is considered as an important aspect of all patellar dysfunctions.

PATELLAR DISLOCATION

In normal motion of gliding in the patellar groove of the distal anterior aspect of the femur the patella is dependent upon the tendinous aspect of the quadriceps mechanism, the depth of the groove, its own intrinsic structure, and the alignment of the entire musculoskeletal components of the lower extremity.

In review of anatomy the patella has a smooth posterior articulating surface that is covered with cartilage and presents two facets divided by a vertical ridge that fits into a corresponding groove between the two condyles of the femur.

Dislocation in which the patella leaves its femoropatellar groove can occur for various reasons. An acute injury or violent stress can cause dislocation of an otherwise normal patella. Such insults occur from severe falls or external injuries, such as auto accidents or athletic injuries with violent lateral rotatory stress imposed upon the knee on the weight-bearing leg.

Dislocation can be present in the newborn as a congenital abnormality. The patella may be poorly formed, the femoropatellar groove inadequate, or the alignment faulty because of severe varus or valgus knee. Diagnosis in the newborn usually is made by clinical examination because x-ray film of the knee fails to reveal the patella, which does not ossify until age two to six. Correction of the genu valgus is usually considered in the newborn.

73

An acute dislocation can predispose the knee to further episodes. Other factors can exist that predispose dislocation from minor stress upon the knee (Fig. 52). These include:

1. Marked genu valgum that laterally displaces the patella or improperly aligns the extensor mechanism.
2. An elongated patellar tendon that causes a slack in the patellofemoral junction.
3. A deficient vastus medialis.
4. External tibial torsion.
5. A shallow patellar groove on the femur.
6. A lateral patellar attachment on the tubercle.
7. A shallow lateral femoral condyle.
8. A deformed patella.

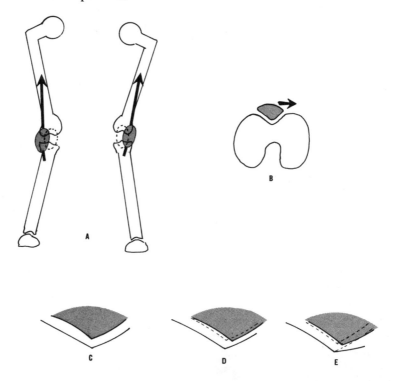

FIGURE 52. Mechanism of patellar dislocation. *A*, Legs with lateral deviation and stress upon the patella in genu valgus. The arrow depicts the direction of stress. *B*, Skyline view; *C*, Normal patellofemoral articulation; *D*, Normal concave patellar lateral facet with a smaller convex medial facet; *E*, Flattened shallower femoral condyle. Either the lateral or the medial facets and/or condyles can be defective.

74

One of the first symptoms is a tendency for the knee to buckle, causing the patient to fall or lose his balance. Pain and tenderness over the anterior knee area follows. Effusion is frequent but is not as severe as in an internal knee injury. There may be some difficulty in extending the knee but when extension is accomplished, either actively or passively, the patella returns to its normal position.

Examination reveals one or more of the contributing factors listed above. There is usually excessive laxity of the extensor mechanism and excessive movement of the patella is possible generally in a lateral direction. The vastus medialis may be atrophic. Crepitation is felt and heard between the patella and its femoral groove. X-ray studies in the adult may reveal a malformed patella, a shallow femoral condyle, or merely a faulty position of the patella as compared to the normal side. In cases of recurrent dislocation chondromalacia patellae may be evident.

A recurrent dislocating patella frequently occurs as an associated condition of other knee joint pathology that impairs the extensor mechanism, such as the narrowing of the knee joint space, malalignment from meniscus disease, or degenerative arthritis.

There are many types of treatment advocated, evidence that no one form of treatment has proven to be completely effective. Repair is aimed at changing the line of quadriceps pull, restoring the depth of the femoral sulcus, or decreasing the quadriceps laxity. In severe patellar dislocation in which the paripatellar reticulum is torn surgical repair is indicated.

PATELLAR FRACTURE

Fracture is frequent because of the exposed position of the patella and the severe stress imposed upon it in violent activities. Trauma is thus direct or indirect. Diagnosis should pose no problem if a fractured condition is suspected. The history may include a blow to the knee or a fall upon the patella (direct). In older, usually obese and deconditioned individuals, indirect injury is elicited by a history of a jump, descending the stairs, a forceful squat, etc. with an audible and painful snap followed by fall or loss of balance. Usually the patient then is unable to extend the knee.

Examination reveals swelling about the patella, tenderness, and usually some effusion. The appearance of the patella may reveal deformity and occasionally fragments of the patella may

75

be movable manually by the examiner. X-ray pictures are helpful in diagnosis.

Treatment may present problems but a cardinal rule exists: *the patella must be conserved if at all possible.* The concept that the patella is of no value to knee extensor function is not tenable. Excision of the patella is considered only when there has been severe comminution leaving no single fragment of significant size to be of value to the extensor mechanism.

Therefore, treatment may be conservative or surgical. In the conservative approach, effusion, and especially hemarthrosis, must be aspirated, repeatedly if necessary. A posterior mold splint that fully extends the knee is applied and the knee is packed in ice for several days until all swelling is eliminated. Then a skin-tight cast is applied, and replaced as needed to maintain firm contact, for a period of 4 to 8 weeks. Crutch walking is permitted. Quadriceps setting exercises are begun early and carefully supervised to secure maintenance of quadriceps strength.

Surgical intervention requires good judgment by an experienced orthopedic surgeon. Surgery involves:

1. Replacement and fixation of the fragments.
2. Removal of entire patellar fragments. (Total or partial patellectomy as treatment of patellar fractures has resulted in good functional recovery with no adverse effect on knee motion, strength, or stability (Mishra). Complete excision is not usually followed by femoral condyle arthritic change nor ossification of the patellar tendon.)
3. Removal of all fragments, leaving only an adequate large fragment.
4. Replacement of the patella with a prosthesis.

Realignment of fragments with fixation is usually unsuccessful because congruity of the articular surface is not attainable and cannot be maintained against the forceful traction of the quadriceps and the poor osteogenesis of the patella. Nonunion of fragments or chondromalacia patellae is a fragment result. Good results from internal fixation usually exist where there are two equal fragments that approximate anatomically. Best results are reported when one large fragment can be salvaged and all other fragments removed.

Osteochondral fractures must be considered when x-ray studies fail to reveal any abnormality but clinical suspicion exists and when the history and symptoms are similiar to that of a patellar fracture.

The history is usually of a teenager or young adult who sustains direct or indirect trauma, which he causes by twisting or jumping on a flexed, weight-bearing knee, thus giving rise to a lateral dislocation of the patella. An osteochondral fracture may result with or without a resultant loose body. Medial tenderness is elicited and the hemarthrosis may reveal flecks of fat in the aspirated fluid. X-rays may reveal the loose body. Arthrography (see Chapter 3) may be necessary for diagnosis and, if available, should precede diagnostic arthrotomy.

Conservative treatment as mentioned in fractures is indicated, but surgical exploration is valid when symptoms are persistent or of greater severity than expected from examination and x-ray studies.

CHONDROMALACIA PATELLAE

This term is used to denote a condition of pain arising from cartilaginous abnormality of the posterior aspect of the patella. Trauma has been implicated but the exact cause remains unanswered. Patients are usually young individuals, a fact which may indicate existence of constitutional factors. Repeated minor traumata may cause cartilage infraction and disturb the nutrition of the cartilage with gradual progressive degenerative changes. The first changes are those of swelling followed by dessication, thinning, and ultimately fissuring and erosion.

The degree of chondromalacia has been graded:

I: Localized softening, swelling, and fibrillation of the cartilage.
II: Fragmentation and fissuring of an area 1.3 cm. or less in diameter.
III: Fragmentation and fissuring of an area more than 1.3 cm. in diameter.
IV: Erosion of cartilage down to subchondral bone. In advanced cases the opposing femoral cartilage area is also affected.

Studies done on normal knees have revealed a surprisingly large number of asymptomatic chondromalacia cartilages. Similiar studies have found abnormal cartilages with increasing frequency as age increased, with indications that changes begin usually at 20 years of age and are found in nearly everyone at 35.

A mechanical etiological factor is implied in the finding of a ridge on the femoral condyle, the ridge more often being medial than lateral (Fig. 53). Incongruity of the patellofemoral articulation has also been described (Wiberg) (Fig. 54). Excess weight has been incriminated as well as abnormal length of the patellar tendon.

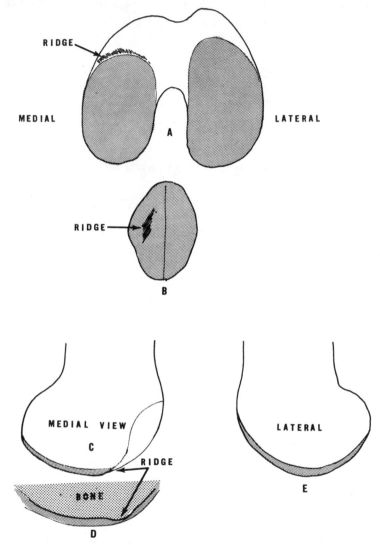

FIGURE 53. Ridge concept of chondromalacia patellae. *A,* A ridge has been discovered to exist at the anterior border of the medial femoral condyle, which causes erosion upon the patella, *B. C,* A lateral view of the site of the ridge, which apparently is a ledge of bone, *D,* underlying the cartilage. No similar ridge exists on the lateral condyle, *E.*

In advanced cases the opposing femoral cartilage area is also affected. Recent studies have revealed hyperplasia of chondrocytes, new bone formation, and thinning of the subchondral osseous plate with severe osteoporosis of the trabecular bone. The osteoporosis seems to imply an intrinsic causation of chondromalacia patellae rather than its being secondary to osteoarthrosis or primary degeneration of the cartilage. Much further research needs to be done.

Among the symptoms are those of retropatellar aching that may be described by the patients as giving way or locking but these rarely occur. There is complaint of stiffness after prolonged sitting and crepitation may be felt or heard. Pain is related to quadriceps contraction and is noted in climbing stairs or arising from a chair.

Examination usually reveals a normal knee. Testing by having the patient climb up on a step or a stool with resultant pain in the patellar region is suggestive. Tenderness over the medial aspect may be elicited. Pain and crepitation occurs from pressure against the patella or downward resistance upon the patella during a forceful quadriceps contraction. Effusion is rare and the knee is stable. X-ray results in the early stages are negative. In advanced cases lateral x-ray views may show an irregular posterior surface or marginal osteophytes. Arthrograms are normal except in advanced cases.

Treatment is variable but should be conservative until disability and severity dictates otherwise. Some physicians elect retropatellar steroid injections. Knee flexion should be avoided,

FIGURE 54. Mechanism of chondromalacia caused by the femoral condylar ridge. As the knee flexes the patella is dragged across the ridge (see Fig. 53) and irritates the patellar cartilage. The irritation occurs between 15° and 30° of flexion.

79

especially weight-bearing flexion. This may require the application of a cylindrical cast.

As restricted activities continue quadriceps exercises should be initiated to prevent quadriceps atrophy and instability. Isometric (setting) exercises rather than range of motion isotonic exercises are better tolerated by the patient but should be performed by gradually extending the knee until the patella is fully elevated cephalad with the knee fully extended before maximum contracture is done. This minimizes the motion of the patella.

The patellofemoral joint reaction force is 3.3 times body weight during stair climbing and 7 times that of level ground walking, which accounts for the increase of pain during activities. Pressure of the patella upon the femoral condyle results from quadriceps tension and is dependent upon the angle of knee flexion. Quadriceps exercises using a 9 kg. boot from 90° flexion to full extension causes 1.4 times the stress imposed by body weight. The greatest stress occurs at 36° of knee flexion. The same exercise done with weighted straight leg raising imposes only 0.5 times the body weight. This explains the reluctance of the patient to do progressive resistance exercises using a heavy boot and moving the knee through complete range of motion.

Surgical intervention varies from arthrotomy with shaving of the involved cartilage or the femoral ridge to ultimately performing a patellectomy. Patellectomy would be a more acceptable treatment if the condition of all patients inevitably deteriorated, but the natural history of this affliction is that of usual improvement to an asymptomatic status.

OSGOOD-SCHLATTER'S DISEASE

This condition is osteochondritis of the tibial tubercle. It is observed in adolescents, usually boys, and frequently is bilateral. The onset is insidious. The patient is aware of pain and tenderness over the tibial tubercle. The condition is aggravated by exercise or from direct pressure such as kneeling. Swelling of the tubercle or the tendon where it attaches to the tubercle is noted.

During adolescence the attachment of the tubercle to the tibial shaft is a weak link of the quadriceps mechanism. Repeated traction stresses predispose to minor avulsion of the ossification center. These changes are similar to those described in Larsen-Johannson's disease of the patella.

A theory has been postulated that bony changes are actually secondary to swelling, hemorrhage, and degenerative changes of the patellar tendon near its attachment. These changes in the tendon impair the circulation of the underlying bone and cause irregular ossification. The ossification irregularities appear months after subsistence of the tendon swelling. Nature repairs the irregularity years after the onset.

The only abnormality noted clinically is swelling of the patellar tendon and some swelling of the tubercle with tenderness on pressure and from resisted quadriceps contraction. X-ray studies are negative early in the disease.

Usually treatment is merely avoidance of excessive activity such as running and jumping, knee flexion, and kneeling. If the condition is more severe a cylindrical cast may be applied to the extended knee for several weeks to two months. Rarely is surgery considered. Such surgery consists of tendon splitting, multiple drilling of the tubercle, or bone grafting.

LARSEN-JOHANNSON'S DISEASE

This is an osteochondritis condition affecting the poles of the patella, most often the inferior pole. This condition, and supposedly the etiology, is similiar to Osgood-Schlatter's disease of the tibial tubercle. It also is noted in adolescents, usually boys, with insidious onset of pain, tenderness, and some swelling over the inferior pole of the patella. The condition is aggravated by exercise or any activity that places stress on the patellar tendon. In early stages there are no bony changes noted on x-ray films but later an irregularity may be seen at the inferior pole.

Treatment consists of avoidance of activities by application of a cast if necessary. Usually 6 to 8 weeks of inactivity eliminates the symptoms.

OSTEOCHONDRITIS DISSECANS

This is a painful knee condition in which a fragment of articular cartilage with some subchondral bone separates partially or completely from the joint surface. The latter becomes a foreign body in the joint. It occurs in children, as an anomaly of ossification in adolescents (juvenile osteochondritis), or in adults. Males are most commonly affected.

Onset is usually insidious with pain described as aching and

81

FIGURE 55. Sites of osteochondritis dissecans of the knee. *Above*, Most (85%) occur on the medial femoral condyle; *A*, Classical with 69% on the lateral border of the medial condyle; *B*, Extended classical with 6%; *C*, An inferiocentral site with 10%. *Below*, 15% occur on the lateral condyle; *D*, inferiocentral with 13%; *E*, An anterior site with 2%.

FIGURE 56. An x-ray skyline view for visualizing the femoral condyles.

poorly localized; stiffness is claimed. When a loose body is present in the joint the knee can lock. Incidents of the knee giving way are frequent. This symptom is considered as an indication for surgical intervention.

Physical findings are sparce and nonspecific. There may be quadriceps atrophy, deep tenderness over the femoral condyle, and occasionally the loose body can be palpated. Diagnosis is verified by carefully x-raying the knee, with the use of tomograms if necessary.

Etiological factors are:

1. Trauma from contact of the tibial tuberosity while striking the inner aspect of the femoral condyle or from a torn cartilage that narrows the joint.
2. Circulatory obstruction from thrombus or embolus (most unlikely as the condition frequently is bilateral).
3. Endocrine imbalance.
4. Heredity.

Differentiation of anomaly of ossification (at age 10), juvenile osteochondritis (age 15), and osteochondritis dissecans (adult) aids the choice of treatment because time, rest, and immobilization cure the ossification anomaly but not always the other two.

X-ray films are diagnostic in that they indicate the presence of the condition and the site. Special views, such as the so-called tunnel view, are frequently needed. The various types and sites are shown in Figures 55 and 56.

Treatment in very young children consists of immobilization with a cylindrical cast, followed by serial x-ray studies. Surgical intervention consists of excision of the fragment, removal of the foreign body, or nailing of the fragment.

BIBLIOGRAPHY

Aichroth, P.: Osteochondritis dissecans of the knee. J. Bone Joint Surg. [Br] 53:440, 1971.
Bentley, G.: Chondromalacia patellae. J. Bone Joint Surg. [Am] 52:221, 1970.
Cave, E. F., and Rowe, C. R.: The patella: Its importance in derangement of the knee. J. Bone Joint Surg. [Am] 32:542, 1950.
Crooks, L. M,: Chondromalacia patellae: Early results of a conservative operation. J. Bone Joint Surg. [Br] 49:495, 1967.
Darracott, J., and Vernon-Roberts, V.: The bony changes in "chondromalacia patellae." Rheumatol. Phys. Med. 11:175, 1971.
Hollinghead, W. H.: Functional Anatomy of the Limbs and Back, ed. 2. W. B. Saunders Company, Philadephia, 1960.

Kaufer, H.: Mechanical function of the patella. J. Bone Joint Surg. [Am] 53:1551, 1971.

Mishra, U. S.: Late results of patellectomy in fractured patella. Acta Orthop. Scand. 43:256, 1972.

Osgood, R. B.: Lesions of tibial tubercle occurring during adolescence. Boston M. S. J. 148:114, 1903.

Outerbridge, R. E.: Further studies on the etiology of chondromalacia patellae. J. Bone Joint Surg. [Br] 46:179, 1964.

Outerbridge, R. E.: The etiology of chondromalacia patellae. J. Bone Joint Surg. [Br] 43:752, 1961.

Reilly, D. T., and Martens, M.: Experimental analysis of the quadriceps muscle force and patello-femoral joint reaction force for various activities. Acta Orthop. Scand. 43:126, 1972.

Smillie, I. S.: Osteochondritis dissecans of the knee. Am. J. Orthop. 6:236, 1964.

Wiberg, G.: Spontaneous healing of osteochondritis dissecans in the knee joint. Acta Orthop. Scand. 14:270, 1943.

Wiberg, G.: Roentgenographic and anatomic studies on the patellofemoral joint with special reference to chondromalacia patellae. Acta Orthop. Scand. 12:319, 1941.

Wilpulla, E., and Vahvanen, V.: Chondromalacia of the patellae. Acta Orthop. Scand. 42:521, 1971.

CHAPTER 6

Arthritides Affecting the Knee

RHEUMATOID ARTHRITIS

It is not the intent here to discuss arthritis in all its aspects: nomenclatures, classifications, etiologies, theories, and all their ramifications. These are the bases of large volumes and numerous articles and constitute the life studies of many authors. It is the purpose here to summarize that which is considered factual of the more prevalent types of arthritis, as they relate to the knee joint, for the purpose of diagnosis and better medical and surgical management.

Rheumatoid disease is a systemic disease: an inflammatory disorder of connective tissue with primary involvement of synovial membranes. Some organs of parenchymal tissue are involved as well as small arteries. Consideration here will be confined to the joints, tendons and their sheaths, and capsules (Fig. 57). The synovial tissues have limited ability to react and do so in a nonspecific manner. Rheumatoid disease does not elicit a specific pathognomic or diagnostic type of inflammation. The diagnosis of rheumatoid disease is thus possible on clinical ground with confirmation by laboratory tests. The criteria for diagnosis has been postulated by the American Rheumatism Association to include (1) morning stiffness, (2) pain on motion of joints, (3) symmetrical swelling of joints, (4) subcutaneous nodules, (5) typical changes seen on x-ray film, and (6) positive test for rheumatoid factor. Further revisions of these criteria are constantly under study.

Rheumatoid inflammation begins as congestion, edema, and cellular infiltration with plasma cella and lymphocytes predominating; in the acute phase there may be a large proportion of polymorphs present. In the early phase of the disease the joint surface may be covered with fibrinoid material while fibroblasts and capillaries invade the synovial tissue. This latter activity thickens the inflamed tissue and tends to organize the fibrinous tissue. The synovial fluid simultaneously undergoes inflammatory reaction. The surrounding joint capsule and contiguous tendons and ligaments also undergo inflammatory reactions that, to this date being nonspecific, are considered to be physicochemical.

As the process continues, marginal erosions occur in the subchondral bone and the cartilage undergoes degenerative changes and pannus appears (Fig. 58).

Pannus is an apron of vascular granulation tissue consisting of proliferating fibroblasts, collagen fibers, small blood vessels, and numerous inflammatory cells. The current concept of articular damage and pannus formation is no longer considered to be cartilage destruction by the pannus but rather that cartilage destruction precedes pannus formation. Joints of acute rheumatoid arthritis of several weeks' duration have revealed articular matrix depletion and *no* pannus formation. There has even been expressed the opinion that the pannus does not *invade* the cartilage but rather that it is formed from conversion of cartilage into

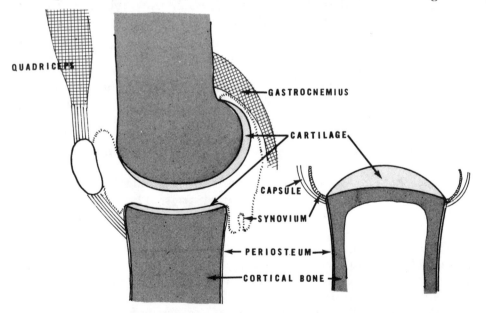

FIGURE 57.   Knee joint structures: schematic. *Left,* Structures forming the joint; *Right,* Graphic illustration of the relationship of the capsule and the synovial membrane to the cartilaginous-cortical union.

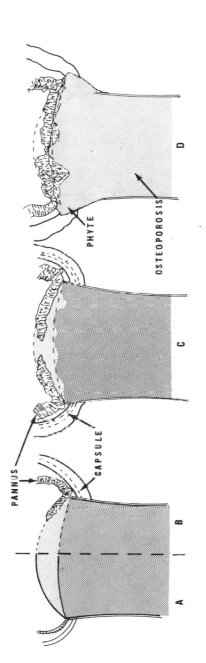

FIGURE 58. Progressive stages of rheumatoid disease of a joint. *A*, The normal half of a joint; *B*, Early thickening of the synovium, caused by edema, congestion, and invasion of fibroblasts and capillaries. The thickened synovium becomes termed pannus and gradually covers the cartilage. The capsule thickens. *C*, Pannus gradually invades and replaces the cartilage and the subchondral bone undergoes erosion. *D*, Advanced stage of the disease with loss of cartilage replaced by fibrous pannus, erosion of the subchondral bone, osteophyte (marginal) formation, and osteoporosis of the cortex. Only one bone that forms the joint has been shown, but the same condition is occurring in all the bones of the joint simultaneously.

fibrous tissue by metamorphosis of chondrocytes into fibroblasts. The exact mechanism of cartilage destruction is not known.

The interface between the pannus and the cartilage has been found to be crossed by fine collagen fibers, which may indicate that the pannus is not the destructive agent but rather is engaged in repairing the damaged cartilage with fibrous tissue. There are recent studies (Mills) that indicate that the granulation tissue that replaces the damaged cartilage is *not* a direct extension of synovium but rather is invasion from the subchondral vascular spaces and from the marrow through the subchondral bone plate (Fig. 59). Pannus formation is considered to be a late phenomenon following the subchondral invasion. Synovial disease must initiate the process with all subsequent reactions being secondary.

Normally the cartilage matrix consists of water, collagen, and protein polysaccharides. It is thought that the chondrocyte secretes the matrix, thus providing the rigidity and elasticity of the cartilage. The matrix is traversed by crisscrossing fibrils. The matrix has a limited life span and must be constantly renewed by the chondrocytes. Rheumatoid arthritis may arise from impairment of chondrocyte function as it furnishes the matrix (Fig. 60).

Lysosomes that contain enzymes capable of degrading all types of macromolecules (proteinases for proteins, carbohydrases, and lipases) are well surrounded by a membrane that

FIGURE 59.   Schematic route of articular disease. *F*, The fibrinoid film that covers the cartilage and ultimately undergoes organization. *P*, Pannus, which is inflamed synovium that contains fibroblasts and capillaries. It has fine collagen fibers connecting to the cartilage. *V*, Deep blood vessels. *M* and *C*, Marrow and cortex invasion of osteoclasts that penetrate the subcortical bone plate to invade the cartilage and ultimately destroy it from within.

holds in the enzymes. In rheumatoid disease a *factor* is released, which possibly ruptures the membrane and releases the enzymes that attack the chondrocytes. The factor possibly is chemical, an immunoglobulin, but presently is unknown. Rheumatoid disease also releases *fibrin*, a protein that may line the cartilage surface and deny entrance of the necessary nutrients.

Rheumatoid disease is currently considered to be an antigen-antibody reaction initiated by a bacterial or viral organism. It is this antigen-antibody reaction that releases the lysosome enzymes (see Fig. 60).

As the joint narrows from cartilage resorption the subchondral bone has and is undergoing erosion (see Fig. 58) with ultimate osteophyte formation at the margins. There is subsequent capsular thickening which combines with the fibrous replacement of the cartilage.

The ultimate stage of rheumatoid disease of the joint is

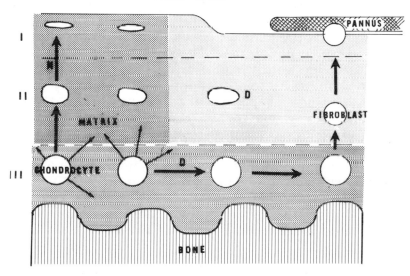

FIGURE 60. Schematic of theory of cartilage degradation in rheumatoid arthritis. The chondrocytes, located in the basal layers, *III*, secrete the matrix (primarily water, collagen, and protein polysaccharides). As the chondrocyte ages it migrates, *arrows*, towards the joint space, *N*. As degradation, *D*, occurs (cause unknown) the intermediate zone, *II*, loses metachromatic mucopolysaccharide (stains alkaline). A theory is expounded which claims that some chondrocytes become fibroblasts that migrate peripherally to form the pannus. The pannus consists of vascular granulating tissue, proliferating fibroblasts, inflammatory cells, and collagen fibers. The chondrocytes may begin degradation when they are attacked by enzymes liberated from the lysosomes, which in turn were damaged by an infectious agent: virus, bacteria, etc.

89

either fibrous ankylosis or osteoarthritic degeneration with loss of all joint motion. The disease process may continue to ultimate destruction or stop at any stage, undergo some remission, have recurrences, or be aborted early before any destructive changes are evident.

History and Examination

The usual age of onset of this rheumatoid disease is between 20 and 40 years, but there is a childhood form of the disease known as Still's disease, and onset has even been recorded in the sixth decade. The joints most frequently involved early in the disease are the hands and feet with the involvement being polyarticular and bilateral. In subsequent frequency of incidence come the wrists, ankles, elbows, and knees. Females are afflicted twice as often as males.

The disease is systemic. The patient appears ill, fatigues easily, and has poor appetite and poor nutrition. Anemia is prevalent. The patient is apprehensive and exhibits signs of vasomotor instability and poor muscle tone. The involved joints are swollen, warm, and tender, and palpation reveals swelling with a peri-articular bogginess. All joint motions (both active and passive) are avoided because of the pain that motion incites. Muscular atrophy is early and marked, as a manifestation of both the associated myopathic component of the disease and the disuse from pain, spasm, and ultimate articular contracture.

The onset systemically may be acute and fulminating or it may be insidious with slow gradual progression and occasional remission and recurrence. The type of disease progress cannot be predicted during the initial episode and no cause of exacerbation after a remission is known. The factors of fatigue, deconditioning, stress, and intercurrent infection have all been implicated.

Laboratory confirmation of the disease is made from elevation of the sedimentation rate: leukopenia (below 5000) is frequent but when there is leukocytosis there is predominace of lymphocytes. Hypoproteinemia occurs and the titer of rheumatoid factors is elevated.

Usually the disease has been clinically evident and diagnosed before it is apparent that the knees are the principally involved joints. Synovial fluid drawn from the knee effusion is turbid with elevated specific gravity, slightly decreased sugar, and increase of cellular inclusion (usually polymorphs).

The disease follows a sequence of pathological events (Fig. 61) in which all the tissues of and about the joint are involved simultaneously.

Phase I: Soft tissue involvement. This is primarily synovial hyperemia with joint effusion. The surrounding ligaments and capsule are stretched, swollen, and tender. X-ray pictures tak-

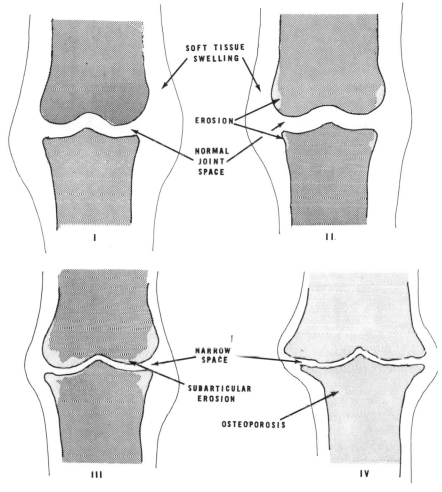

FIGURE 61.   Changes in rheumatoid arthritis seen by X ray. *Phase I,* Early signs reveal soft tissue swelling with a normal joint space. Occasionally the swelling may separate the involved joint. *Phase II,* As the disease progresses some erosion is noted at the lateral margins where the collateral ligaments attach. *Phase III,* The erosion spreads centrally to the subchondral region, and the joint space narrows. *Phase IV,* The joint space becomes occluded as the cartilage completely disappears and bone opposes bone; the capsule is now fibrotic and not swollen (effused). There are bilateral osteophytes.

en at this stage merely reveal the soft tissue swelling with no articular changes.

Phase II: Continuation of synovitis, now with pannus formation and evidence of *nonarticular* bone destruction. It is at this stage that the synovium begins invasion of the cartilage and the adjacent bone. X-ray pictures here become diagnostic as there is noticable bone destruction (erosion) at the margins of the articular cartilage under the collateral ligaments and appearance of decalcification. The joint space remains intact on routine x-ray study but arthroscopy would reveal the presence of pannus and some erosion of cartilage.

Phase III: Destruction of the cartilage and subchondral bone erosion. The joint space is now narrower; this is most apparent on the lateral aspect of the joint. Instability of the knee is now apparent. Soft tissue swelling has lessened because the synovial tissue is now more fibrotic and less inflamed and vascular. The periarticular swelling is firmer and feels thicker.

Phase IV: Joint destruction of varying degree with marked cartilage destruction, which is apparent on x-ray film. There is marked joint laxity through ligamentous involvement which causes slackness as a result of the joint space narrowing.

Treatment

Treatment demands symptomatic medical treatment of rheumatoid disease; this will not be discussed in detail here. Suffice it to say that, in addition to a high protein diet, medication consists of salicylates, phenylbutazone, antimalarial drugs, gold salts, and steroids, dependent upon the experience of the treating physician. None as yet are specific. There are advocates of intra-articular injection of long-acting steroids. However, since this disease is prone to chronicity and recurrence and because repeated intra-articular steroids have been implicated in steroid arthropathy, the repeated use of steroids is not recommended as routine treatment.

Treatment of the knee afflicted with rheumatoid arthritis consists of physical methods with prevention of deformity as the goal. Unlike other joints that may be involved and for which complete *rest* of prolonged duration is valuable this tenet of complete rest and immobilization is not plausible in the knee. Flexion contraction, quadriceps atrophy, fibrous adhesions with possible ankylosis, and subluxation are frequent and severe; once established they are resistant to treatment. Reversibility of pathological changes is difficult and often impossible.

Exercise: The position of flexion must be avoided during the acute phase. Unfortunately this is the position of comfort to the patient; it is promoted by musclar spasm as well as joint capsular inflammation. Pillows must not be permitted under the knee during bedrest. Posterior mold splints can be made both to protect the extended knee and to afford comfort. The leg must be exercised periodically while in the splints. This can be done by assisted removal of the leg from the splint and gentle active and passive flexing and extending of the knee several times daily. This routine prevents intra-articular fibrosis and capsular contracture. Heat or ice applications as tolerated by the patient should accompany this daily ritual.

The quadriceps must be exercised immediately and frequently and with effort in this disease. The type of exercise best tolerated in the *acute* joint phase is that of quadriceps setting (isometric) straight leg raising within the cast and during the period when the cast is removed. A gradual increase of this quadriceps activity to active isotonic resisted exercises should be made as tolerated. Weight bearing should be avoided except with the aid of crutches or walker and should be strictly avoided if any flexion contracture exists. Use of braces or cages, which immobilize the extended knee, is to be discouraged because it adds to further atrophy and dependence.

Upon subsidence or decrease of inflammation with its resultant spasm and painful joint motion, active exercises should be instituted. These are similar to the exercises described in Chapter 3. Once resistive exercises are initiated they should be carefully supervised, done frequently during the day, and gradually *increased with encouragement.* Patient fear and low threshold of pain are strong factors which delay progress in rehabilitation efforts. Fear that pain means aggravation of the disease must be allayed and constant encouragement should be given. After remission or subsidence of the acute phase of the illness a progressive exercise program must be maintained in order to minimize any possible exacerbation that, being superimposed on a partial residual disability, could have detrimental disabling effects.

Aspiration. During the acute stages of phase *I* or *II* significant effusion should be aspirated because its persistence will over-distend the capsule and ligaments and limit range of joint motion. Passive and active exercises during effusion are limited.

The technique of intra-articular aspiration is relatively simple but justifies clarification. Asceptic conditions are mandatory because an arthritic joint with superimposed infection can be calamitous.

93

Entrance preferably is made from the lateral side. The patella is passively moved towards the lateral side, which widens the joint space between the patella and the femoral condyle (Fig. 62).

Normally there is insufficient synovial fluid to aspirate. In effusion or hemarthrosis the leg can be placed with the lateral margin down. This can be accomplished by laterally rotating the reclining patient. Gravity causes the fluid to seek a dependent position. An 18 gauge needle is inserted into the suprapatellar pouch. By also injecting air (approximately 10 cc.) and then applying manual pressure in the popliteal space the fluid is further brought to the needle. The needle can be withdrawn slowly while aspirating to completely evacuate the fluid.

The initial tapped fluid should be studied for cell count, presence of crystals, sugar, mucin, and other pertinent diagnos-

FIGURE 62.   Aspiration of the knee joint. *A*, Technique of laterally moving the patella, *P*, to increase the injectable space between the patella and the femoral condyle. *B*, Lateral view, *black dot*, site of injection and P_p, popliteal space pressure to bring fluid to needle tip. *C*, With lateral position the fluid gravitates to permit easier aspiration.

tic studies. Intra-articular steroids at the time of aspiration is questionable since the benefit is not fully accepted and the detrimental effect of intra-articular steroids, especially if repeated, is well documented.

Surgery. Findings that indicate continued active synovitis and persistence of symptoms *after six months* (arbitrarily determined) indicate the desirability of synovectomy. The efficacy of synovectomy has not been proven in halting the systemic ravages of the disease nor in preventing recurrences. However, it is an accepted fact that synovectomy does delay damage to the articular cartilage, may initiate a remission of the disease, and possibly decreases the synovial reaction of other joints simultaneously affected. Synovectomy does *not* damage an intact joint and it does prevent phase I of the rheumatoid joint from advancing into phase II and III.

Synovectomy in phase III probably does not decrease further degenerative changes but does aid in joint management when performed also for the sake of debridement. In phase III careful consideration must be given regarding arthroplasty prosthesis. At this date the devices used are the McIntosh or McKeever prostheses or the femoral condyle prosthesis of Aufranc. Total knee replacements have not been proven in the number done and duration of their use to be recommended.

The aim of arthroplasty is to alleviate pain, correct deformity, and increase joint range of motion. Hemiarthrodesis aims to correct a varus or valgus deformity (Fig. 63). A tibial plateau prosthesis of proper width realigns the joint, creates a smooth painless gliding surface and adheres to the tibia by virtue of its serrated undersurface. When the joint is physiologically realigned the ligaments resume their normal length. The collateral ligaments do not lose their normal length in long-standing varus or valgus deformity. Prosthesis should be considered *only* when synovectomy, debridement, or tibial osteotomy have been considered and found of no value or when there is no remaining cartilage and bone is rubbing against bone. The prosthesis becomes covered with a layer of fibrous tissue that forms an envelope around it and helps bind it down. Postoperative success may depend on this development.

Prostheses are contraindicated when there has been a previous plateau fracture or previous infection or fusion, when a neurotrophic arthritis exists, or when there is questionable patient cooperation. Severe joint destruction may be a contraindication; arthroscopy here may help verify the existence of remaining cartilage.

Arthrodesis will provide a stable and pain-free knee; it is a salvage operation that is considered the final solution. However, recommendation of this procedure depends on the condition of the other joint of the extremity and the ability of the patient to function adequately with the other knee. Preoperatively the involved knee can be temporarily immobilized by casting as a test of the patient's functional ability and acceptance of the inability to flex the knee. Further involvement of the remaining uninvolved knee may cause irreversible disability and precludes other surgery short of total knee replacement.

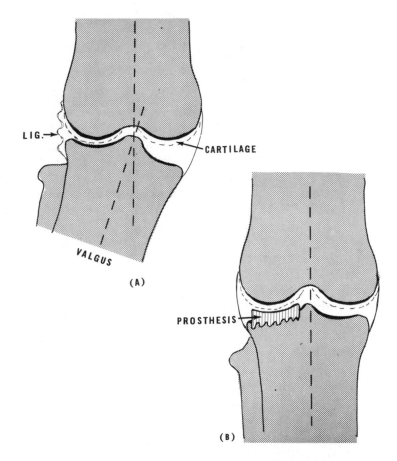

FIGURE 63.   Treatment of degenerative arthritis with tibial plateau hemiprosthesis. *A*, The usual valgus of the degenerated knee joint with marked narrowing of the lateral joint compartment. The capsule is redundant. *B*, Insert of the prosthesis straightens the knee and separates the lateral joint space.

Osteoarthritis, also commonly called degenerative arthritis or osteoarthrosis, connotes joint disease that is degenerative as compared to inflammatory or infectious. It is thus differentiated from rheumatoid arthritis and its variants. Osteoarthritis is differentiated as primary (idiopathic) or secondary to a preceding infectious, traumatic, inflammatory, metabolic, or aging process. Regardless of classification the pathomechanics of the joint disease is not known.

Osteoarthritis is essentially a degenerative condition of the joint articular cartilage with subsequent formation of marginal osteophytes, subchondral bone changes, bone marrow changes, fibrous reaction of the synovium, and capsular thickening.

Early degenerative changes may be asymptomatic until synovitis develops with effusion, stiffness, capsular thickening, and formation of marginal osteophytes. Pain is considered to be caused by the stretching of the periosteum by the expanding osteophytes, bony changes at points of ligamentous attachment, and the protective muscle spasm that occurs to immobilize the painful joint.

Certain changes occur in aging of articular cartilage that are difficult to differentiate from osteoarthritic changes. These changes differ from person to person, joint to joint, and from various areas of the opposing articular surfaces. There are generalized changes in the joint destructive process as well as focal cartilage changes. Normal joints undergo *maturation* that defies differentiation from degenerative changes. Joints are constantly undergoing normal remodeling, a process of wear and repair which is considered to be a destructive process when an imbalance occurs between destruction and repair.

Of the many concepts considered to be causative factors in osteoarthritis the most attractive and acceptable is that which postulates that synovitis represents chronic chemical inflammation of the cartilage resulting from excessive concentration of polysaccharides formed in the joint from debris of damaged cartilage (Fig. 64). This theory has been reproduced experimentally by injecting debris of scraped cartilage intra-articularly with resultant synovitis, capsular thickening, loss of cartilage elasticity (because of loss of protein polysaccharides), fissuring, and ultimate fibrillation with gradual denuding of the cartilage to the depths of subchondral bone.

Fibrillation occurs from vertical fissures, which penetrate to-

97

wards subchondral bone. A loss of mucopolysaccharides may precede or follow the fissuring. The subchondral bone becomes hyperemic and blood vessels containing fibrous tissue penetrate the subchondral plate and enter the denuding cartilage. The idea that metachromatic mucopolysaccharide loss is greatest in the midtransitional zone of the cartilage implies enzymic penetration rather than surface friction as the cause of wear and tear. A proteolytic (collagenase) enzyme appears to be the causative factor.

Salicylates act as an enzyme inhibitor that prevents chondromalacia. This has been documented both clinically and experimentally and when given early and in adequate doses prevents fibrillation. Once fibrillation is established salicylates are ineffective. This fact and other studies indicate that chemical as well as mechanical factors play a major part in osteoarthritis.

Treatment of degenerative arthritis is not complicated but requires attention to details. Mere control of the inflammatory state may leave an unstable knee joint. Heat application is usually beneficial in this type of arthritis and may be applied by hot moist packs, diathermy, or a baker. Weight reduction is mandatory. Evaluation of the patient's daily activities must be thoroughly studied and necessary changes made. Low chairs must be avoided and patient must not remain in the same position for prolonged periods of time. Upon awakening in the morning active flexion and extension of the knee should be done before weight bearing is attempted.

Walking should be encouraged for daily activities but not

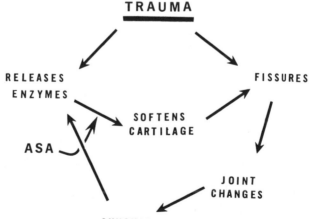

FIGURE 64. Schematic process in progress of degenerative arthritis: site of salicylate action.

forced for the sake of prolonged exercise as a therapy. Deep knee bends also should be avoided. Faulty posture that places a strain on the stance should be corrected. Exercises should be a daily ritual to strengthen the quadriceps extensor group by setting exercises increasing to full progressive resistive exercises as tolerated. Hamstring exercises with the patient standing holding on to a dresser or table and flexing the knee twenty times or to the point of fatigue are beneficial. In the same position gastrocnemius-soleus exercises are performed, in which the patient rises on his toes with both feet simultaneously, one foot alternately, and progresses to toe raising from a book placed under the ball of the foot.

If the patient has a severe valgus or varus of the knee with severe narrowing of the joint on the concave side osteotomy of the tibia and fibula can relieve the patient's symptoms by shifting his weight to the opposite side of the joint.

HEMOPHILIC ARTHRITIS

Hemophilia is an abnormal hemorrhaging condition with hereditary and familial tendencies sustained by males and transmitted by females. Essentially the disease is a failure of blood to clot with a resultant period of excessive bleeding. Hemarthrosis, bleeding into the joint, is common and presents a major adversity of the disease with resultant disability.

Onset of hemophilia is usually at 4 to 10 years and is noted initially as a sequela of trauma. The knee, because of its exposure to stress and injury, frequently is involved and hemarthrosis of the knee is often the first evidence of the disease.

Acute hemarthrosis manifests itself by a rapid swelling of the joint, intense pain, and marked muscle spasm. The joint capsule becomes markedly distended with concomitant swelling of the periarticular tissues. The knee is hot and extremely sensitive and rapidly demonstrates a tight, taut skin over the entire joint. Hemorrhage may become so severe as to rupture through the capsule and penetrate the periarticular soft tissue with ecchymosis and even tissue sloughing.

Intra-articular hemorrhage invades all the intra-articular tissues. Besides damage resulting from the intense distension from the blood, the blood elements irritate the synovial membrane from a toxic effect not fully understood. Blood pigments impregnate the synovium, which changes color, texture, and thickness. The synovium may undergo hyperplasia with formation of

99

villi. Usually the first bout(s) of hemarthrosis subside and the synovium returns to its normal state. With repeated episodes the synovium is invaded by fibrous elements, undergoes hypertrophy, and thickens into a hyperplastic tissue.

Repeated hemarthosis ultimately affects the cartilage adversely, possibly by (1) damage as a result of excessive unremittent pressure of the increased synovial fluid, (2) impairment of the nutritive aspect of the synovial fluid, and (3) toxic elements considered to exist in hemophiliac blood. The latter possibility has not been confirmed.

The cartilage thins and ultimately erodes to the subchondral bone (Fig. 65), causing subchondral sclerosis and cysts. These cysts are considered to be hemorrhaging into the bone cortex. They are noted on x-ray pictures and are especially prominent in the region of the tibial plateau.

In chronic cases the entire joint may become obliterated by firm fibrous adhesions extending from the tibial to the femoral condyles. This thick pannus is fibrous tissue that grows from the subchondral bone through the crevices in the cartilage. Fibrous ankylosis may be the inevitable result.

Flexion deformity occurs early in the affected extremity. The distended capsule and the concomitant hamstring spasm tend to flex the knee, which gives some relief of pain to the patient but on the other hand enhances further disability. With recurrent episodes of hemarthrosis the posterior capsule thickens and thus maintains flexion deformity. Ambulation in this flexed knee position places abnormal stress upon the articular tissues and adds to the deformity.

Treatment of hemophilic arthritis of the knee includes treatment of hemophilia as well as care for other hemorrhagic sites, which may have more drastic residual. Immediate administration of plasma products is imperative following diagnosis. These products must be available. A center for treatment of hemophiliacs may exist in the community; its presence should be known. The products currently recommended: for hemophilia A, AHF plasma concentrate or AHF cryoprecipitate; for hemophilia B (PTC or Factor IX deficiency), plasma concentrate if available. Plasma may be used but it is difficult to elevate the

FIGURE 65.   Hemophilic arthritis. *A*, Hemarthrosis with bloody effusion distending the capsule and putting pressure, *arrows*, against the cartilage of the femur and the tibia. *B*, If there is persistence or frequent recurrence of hemarthrosis the cartilage thins. *C*, Chronic stage with fibrous reaction within the bloody effusion, organization of the hemorrhagic effusion, fibrous invasion through the damaged cartilage, and ultimate fibrous ankylosis.

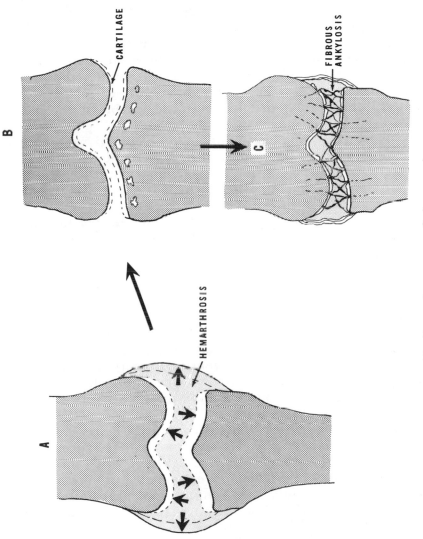

Fɪɢ. 65. (Legend appears on facing page.)

101

AHF level to sufficient hemostatic level with its use. The dosage of plasma products is based on severity of bleeding, patient's weight, thus insuring a minimum of 30 percent AHF or PTC level. Care and good technique in administration are mandatory.

Care of the knee itself is a tedious procedure. Many aspects of treatment may seem feasible yet be instrumental in causing more bleeding. Enforced rest of the knee is mandatory with elevation, cold compresses (possibly ice), and gentle but firm and uniform compression bandaging.

Aspiration of the hemorrhaging articular fluid as an isolated procedure may increase bleeding and therefore must be done after administration of plasma concentrates that raise the level of AHF to 50 percent. It must be done with extreme care of asepsis. Intra-articular instillation of steroid or hyaluronidase has proven to be effective in enhancing absorption of the hemarthrosis, relieving pain simultaneously, and permitting earlier gradual motion. Its instillation into the joint also minimizes the proliferative changes in the synovium, which are the precursor of ulitimate fibrosis. The mode of action of hyaluronidase is not fully understood but it apparently enhances interchange of articular fluid through its effect upon the mucopolysaccharide of the cartilage. It also decreases the viscosity of the synovial fluid and possibly through these and other actions increases the permeability of the synovial membrane.

Hyaluronidase instillation must be aseptically performed. An equal amount of hyaluronidase mixed with 1 percent procaine (or derivative) is added to 4 to 6 cc. of the aspirated fluid and is injected into the joint through the same needle. No further fluid is aspirated. Following the instillation a firm elastic bandage, which exerts uniform, firm but gentle, pressure, is applied and the joint is rested in an elevated position for 24 hours. Persistence of pain and spasm is an indication for a repeat aspiration and instillation in 24 hours.

Pain and swelling usually diminish within 24 hours of the first instillation. In this case a gentle active and passive range of joint motion is encouraged and closely supervised. When the joint is moved frequently with gradual increase of extent there is diminution of fibrosis, capsular thickening, and ultimate ankylosis. Other parenteral and oral antihemorrhagic medications are administered.

With levels of AHF or PTC of 50 percent at the time of aspiration, this procedure can be performed on an outpatient basis. A second dose of plasma concentrate must be given on the fourth or fifth day post-aspiration to assure a level of 20 to 30

102

percent. Twenty-four hours of joint immobilization must be maintained after the aspiration. Some support to the knee may be required for ambulation during the first 24 hours.

Even though elective corrective surgery may now be performed where plasma concentrates are available, the intent is towards prevention of deformity. During the acute phase of hemorrhage the knee can be splinted with a carefully applied well-padded splint with a flexible wire to maintain and increase the range of extension (Fig. 66). The splint may be adjusted daily. A posterior mold splint is effective but must be remade frequently to adjust to the desired angle. Active exercises should be started to maintain or increase quadriceps strength as soon as swelling and pain have subsided. These exercises can be isometric initially with gradual increase to isotonic and resisted.

Retroperitoneal hemorrhage is frequent and may occur in the iliopsoas area, causing femoral nerve damage and hypaesthesia and quadriceps paresis. This should be suspected when there is

FIGURE 66. Corrective splinting of hemophilic arthritis. *1*, During the acute phase of hemarthrosis a splint, consisting of a thigh and a lower leg thermoplastic shell held by Velcro straps, can be connected with a flexible wire that can be bent to gradually extend the knee. The knee is visible and change can be made immediately upon an increase of hemorrhage. *2*, A plaster cast, hinged at the knee, can be made for chronic fibrous contracture of the knee in varying degrees of flexion. Gradual extension is obtained by a dorsal turnbuckle that can be turned gradually several times a day or a few degrees every other day as tolerated.

severe quadriceps weakness and atrophy. Plasma products must be continued to maintain levels of AHF for at least 7 to 10 days. Traction to the hip should *not* be instituted as it may increase bleeding. Quadriceps exercises should be started shortly, preferably in a pool area. Weight bearing should be avoided until hip flexion is less than 25°. If quadriceps paralysis is severe some support may be needed when ambulation is begun.

After fibrous ankylosis to the knee is apparent an active exercise and corrective bracing program (see Fig. 66) usually results in gratifying improvement. If ankylosis is severe and fails to improve, it is generally considered desirable to allow natural ankylosis to occur in the most physiological position rather than attempt surgical arthrodesis.

GOUTY ARTHRITIS

Gout is a hereditary metabolic disease predominantly afflicting males but carried and transmitted by females. Clinically the disease becomes apparent in adult life at age 35 to 50. Many relatives of patients with gout have hyperuricemia but never develop clinical manifestations.

Uric acid is known to be a threshold substance formed by the body, eliminated by the renal glomeruli, circulated in the blood, and reabsorbed partly by the kidney tubules. There are three postulated internal dysfunctions that lead to increased uric acid concentration in tissue fluids:

1. Diminished excretion by the kidneys: decreased glomerular filtration or increased reabsorption by the tubules.
2. Excessive formation of urates as a result of faulty metabolism.
3. Diminished destruction of urates by faulty enzymes.

An excess of urates in the serum does not constitute gout until these urates are deposited into mesenchymal tissues through a chemical or metabolic mechanism. Why and how this alteration of urates occurs is not known. An electrolyte imbalance converting uric acid to a sodium urate is postulated: monosodium urate $(Na (C_5H_3O_3N_4) \bullet H_2O)$.

Urate crystal deposits are prone to develop in avascular rather than vascular tissues, thus its predilection for cartilage, bursae, ligaments, tendons, and epiphysial portions of bone. Tophi (accumulations of urates) are conspicuously absent from muscle, lungs, liver, nervous tissue, and kidneys. Urate crystals are deposited in the superficial layers of the cartilage, causing fibrillation. The cartilage *overlying* the deposit is destroyed (Fig. 67) releasing the crystals into the joint space and into the synovial fluid.

While still within the superficial layers of the cartilage the tophus becomes surrounded by granulation tissue, leukocytes, round cells, and giant cells. There is also surrounding edema and hyperemia. This inflammation and its subsequent emission into the joint fluid softens the tophus. Less than 50 percent of patients with gout exhibit tophi.

During the acute attack a thin pannus forms from the syno-

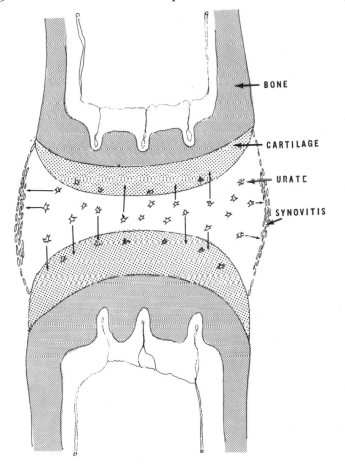

FIGURE 67. Schematic explanation of gouty arthritis. The exact mechanism of gouty arthritis is not verified. The currently accepted theory is that urate crystals form in the synovial fluid and penetrate the outer layer of the cartilage, depositing crystals there. Urate crystals also irritate the synovial layer, causing synovitis. Migration of urates via the subchondral epiphyseal bone is not currently accepted.

vium covering the cartilage surface. There is an increase in synovial fluid and concomitant periarticular inflammation. Clinically the joint is swollen, reddened, and tense with overlying taut, shiny skin. Attack is usually sudden with severely painful swelling and discoloration. Involvement is characteristically in *one* joint, a fact which is of diagnostic significance in differentiating the acute onset of rheumatoid arthritis. The latter is multiarticular and bilateral with symmetrical involvement and usually is found in females or in emaciated sick patients. The acute attack of gout usually subsides within 4 to 7 days leaving a normal joint upon subsidence of the inflammation. Repeated attacks leave permanent damage with joint changes similiar to those noted in osteoarthritis.

Attacks have been considered as resulting from trauma, over-exertion, dietary or alcoholic excesses, surgical procedures elsewhere in the body, or after severe diuresis (usually from use of mercurial salt diuretics).

X-ray studies are not pathognomonic. They reveal similar changes noted in early rheumatoid or degenerative arthritis, but when cysts are noted near the articular margins they are probably masses of urate crystals.

The diagnosis of gouty arthritis consists of a typical history of an acute, *mono*articular, swollen joint with systemic symptoms of fever and leukocytosis. Occurrence is in a male of 35 to 50 years of age in otherwise good health. Uric acid in the serum usually is elevated and crystals may be found in the aspirated joint fluid.

Treatment is prophylactic in regards to systemic treatment. It includes dietary restrictions to avoid purine-rich foods and fats, avoidance of obesity, avoidance of diuretics, and oral administration of colchicine and/or benemid. During the acute episode these drugs, as well as butazolidin or steroids, may be used depending upon the experience of the treating physician.

Care of the involved knee joint is symptomatic. The knee must be immobilized. Effusion, if marked, should be aspirated. A posterior mold splint and cold compresses are effective. Compression dressings usually are poorly tolerated. Recovery after the acute episode is usual with no residual.

PYOGENIC ARTHRITIS

Suppurative arthritis is usually secondary to septicemia or secondary to local invasion. The organism may be identified by joint fluid examination, culture, or blood culture. Treatment demands proper and specific antibiotic administration. Infection into the joint from adjacent bone or soft tissue involvement must be approached by care of that focal point.

The purulent joint must be aspirated (repeatedly if necessary) and antibiotics instilled into the joint as well as given orally or parenterally. The joint must be rested but *flexion must be avoided.* A posterior molded splint may be effective coupled with hot fomentations. Traction is useful to immobilize the knee, maintain adequate extension, and maintain joint surface distraction. As soon as inflammation subsides and allows it, exercise for the quadriceps must be initiated. Ultimately, rehabilitation, as in all arthritides, must be considered.

NEOPLASMS ABOUT THE KNEE

Both primary and metastatic lesions must be considered when pain, deformity, and disability occur in or around the knee joint. Numerous classifications of neoplasms are available in current literature. Diagnosis is made by careful history, taking meticulous examination, x-ray study repeated as often as necessary, isotope scan studies, biopsy, blood chemistry studies, search for primary lesion, etc. Treatment is eventually *the* considered specific treatment for that neoplastic type, extent, duration, and other oncological aspects of the disease.

BURSITIS

Any of the bursae described (see Chapter 1) can become inflamed, swollen, and cause symptoms. Any of these bursae can be swollen and symptomatic or merely noted in the course of routine examination as an asymptomatic swelling. Several types of acute, chronic, or recurrent bursitis about the knee warrant discussion.

The prepatellar bursa lies between the skin and the outer surface of the patella and is prone to direct trauma from a fall or kneeling. Diagnosis from these causes is usually easy with local tenderness, swelling, and inflammation as symptoms. Pain is usually present from tension of the skin in extreme knee flexion or by direct pressure. Treatment for this type of bursitis is usually conservative, it occasionally requires aspiration but rarely does it need incision and drainage. Chronic prepatellar bursitis that results from repeated bouts of irritation may be more recalcitrant to conservative treatment. Drainage followed by pressure dressing and protective padding may be effective. Occasionally total excision of the inflamed thickened bursa is necessary.

Deep infrapatellar bursitis usually occurs from overactivity with undue friction against the upper tibia. This deep bursitis rarely results from direct trauma as the bursa is well protected by the overlying patella and the underlying fat pad. Tenderness can be elicited by pressure *behind* the infrapatellar tendon and from passive forced flexion and active extension of the knee. Treatment is supportive and consists of heat, immobilization, and aspiration. Occasionally instillation of steroids is used but its efficacy is equivocal. Excision is considered when conservative treatment fails.

All other sites of bursitis about the knee usually can be diagnosed by appropriate examination and localizing signs *if bursitis is suspected.*

Posterior bursitis occurs when there are cystic tumors of the popliteal space. The tumors have been termed popliteal or synovial cysts, posterior bursae, Baker's cysts, or semimembranous or gastrocnemius-membranosus bursae. Various authors have claimed from 7 to 50 percent of normal population show communication between the joint space and this posterior popliteal bursa during arthrography. These cysts may include bursal effusion between the medial head of the gastrocnemius and the semimembranosus tendon, which may in turn communicate with the capsule space.

The cause of these popliteal cysts is probably that of normal anatomical connection aggravated by chronic effusion of the intra-articular joint cavity. Chronic effusion may be caused by rheumatoid arthritis, meniscus tear, cruciate ligamentous tears, etc. The incidence of these cysts increase with aging but there is no significant sexual difference.

Treatment of this cyst consists of treatment of the underlying cause. Investigation by arthrography or arthrotomy of any internal articular disease or damage must precede any treatment directed to the cyst. Originally treatment was comprised of excision of the cyst with closure of the communication; this no longer is considered valid in the common cyst. However, if the cyst is large and causing inconvenience it can be aspirated and compressed or it can be totally excised.

BIBLIOGRAPHY

Biggs, R., and MacFarlane, R. G.: Treatment of Hemophilia and Other Coagulation Disorders. F. A. Davis Company, Philadelphia, 1966.

Brattstrom, M.: Asymmetry of ossification and rate of growth of long bones in children with unilateral juvenile gonarthritis. Acta Rheum. Scand. 9:102, 1963.

Byer, P. D.: The pathology of rheumatic diseases, in Licht, Sidney (ed.): Arthritis and Physical Medicine, Ch. 3. Licht, New Haven, 1969.

Campbell, C. J.: The healing of cartilage defects. Clin. Orthop. 64:45, 1969.

Chrisman, O. D.: Biochemical aspects of degenerative joint disease. Clin. Orthop. 64:77, 1969.

Convery, F. R.: The rheumatoid knee. Am. Fam. Physician 4:52, 1971.

Enneking, W. F., and Horowitz, M.: The intra-articular effects of immobilization on the human knee. J. Bone Joint Surg. [Am] 54:973, 1972.

Eyring, E. J.: The therapeutic potential of synovectomy in juvenile rheumatoid arthritis. Arthritis Rheum. 11:688, 1968.

Ghormley, R. K., and Clegg, R. S.: Bone and joint changes in hemophilia. J. Bone Joint Surg. [Am] 30:589, 1948.

Goldie, I., and Schlossman, D.: Radiological changes in rheumatoid knee joints before and after synovectomy Clin. Orthop. 64:98, 1969.

Hall, M. C.: Cartilaginous changes after experimental relief of contact in the knee joint of the mature rat. Clin. Orthop. 64:64, 1969.

Jackson, R. W., and Abe, I.: The role of arthroscopy in management of disorders of the knee. J. Bone Joint Surg. [Br] 54:310, 1972.

Kay, N. R. M., and Martins, H. D.: The MacIntosh tibial plateau hemiprosthesis for the rheumatoid knee. J. Bone Joint Surg. [Br] 54:256, 1972.

MacIntosh, D. L., and Hunter, G. A.: The use of the hemiarthroplasty prosthesis for advanced osteoarthritis and rheumatoid arthritis of the knee. J. Bone Joint Surg. [Br] 54:244, 1972.

Marmor, L.: Osteoarthritis of the knee. J.A.M.A. 218:213, 1971.

Marmor, L.: Surgery of Rheumatoid Arthritis. Henry Kimpton, London, 1967.

Marshall, J. L., and Olson, C. E.: Instability of the knee: A long term experimental study in dogs. J. Bone Joint Surg. [Am] 53:1561, 1971.

McCarty, D. J., Hogan, J. N., Gatten, R., and Grossman, M.: Studies on pathological calcifications in human cartilage. J. Bone Joint Surg. [Am] 48:309, 1966.

McKeever, D. C.: Tibial plateau prosthesis. Clin. Orthop. 18:86, 1960.

McMaster, M.: Synovectomy of the knee in juvenile rheumatoid arthritis. J. Bone Joint Surg. [Br] 54:262, 1972.

Mills, K.: Pathology of the knee joint in rheumatoid arthritis. J. Bone Joint Surg. [Br] 52:746, 1970.

Shands, A. R.: Neuropathies of the bones and joints. Arch Surg. 20:614, 1930.

Sherman, M. S.: The non-specificity of synovial reactions. Bull. Hosp. Jt. Dis. 12:110, 1951.

Smith, C. F., et al.: Long-term management and rehabilitation in hemophilia. Project report, P. H. Grant 110-91. Orthopedic Hospital, Los Angeles, 1969.

Wilson, P. D., Eyre-Brook, A. L., and Francis, J. D.: A clinical and anatomical study of the semimembranosus bursa in relation to popliteal cyst. J. Bone Joint Surg. 20:963, 1938.

Wolfe, R. D., and Colloff, B.: Popliteal cysts. J. Bone Joint Surg. [Am] 54:1057, 1972.

CHAPTER 7

Fractures About the Knee Joint

No treatise of the knee would be complete without discussion of fractures about the knee joint. Some of these fractures may be very complicated and present difficulties in their management, thus full dissertation of all these aspects cannot be covered in this brief monograph. Only basic types and basic principles of their management will be undertaken.

Fractures about the knee may be classified in various categories regarding fractures of the distal end of the femur, proximal end of the tibia, and the patella. Fractures of the distal end of the femur may be divided into supracondylar, intercondylar, and condylar (Fig. 68). Fractures of the tibial plateau may be divided into those (1) involving the lateral condyle or the medial condyle, (2) with or without comminution or displacement, and (3) with variable degrees of depression.

Fractures about the knee must also be evaluated in respect to the injury sustained by the cartilage: chondral fractures involving only the articular cartilage or osteochondral fractures involving the articular cartilage and the underlying subchondral bone. Sudden violent stress can cause avulsion fracture in which a fragment of bone is avulsed by its attachment to a tendon or ligament.

Etiological factors of fractures can be torsion injuries with the fixed foot internally or externally rotated in relationship to the femur, caused by direct violence, or cartilage damage secondary to subluxation of the patella.

Symptoms consist of effusion (hemarthrosis), pain, localized tenderness, crepitation, locking, and varying degrees of disability. X-ray films may be diagnostic but may be unrewarding in chondral fractures. Arthrography may show radiolucent filling defect when a fracture is suspected. Management obviously depends upon the exact mechanism of fracture, the alignment of the fragments, the articular integrity, and proper joint surface alignment. Basic principles must underly all treatment such as removal of fragment, removal of associated meniscus tear, replacement of the fragment with internal fixation, and reconstruction of the extensor mechanism.

FRACTURES OF DISTAL END OF FEMUR

Anatomically the distal end of the femur comprises two large rounded condyles covered with cartilage (see Chapter 1). Muscular attachment about the joint influences the resultant fracture fragments and their alignment. The gastrocnemius muscle pulls the distal fragment posteriorly (Fig. 69) towards the nerves and the blood vessels of the popliteal fossa. The collateral ligaments

FIGURE 68. Fractures about the knee joint: fractures of distal femur and proximal tibia. *1*, Supracondylar fracture; *2*, Intercondylar fracture "Y" type; *3*, Condylar fracture of femur; *4*, Condylar fracture of tibial plateau; *5*, Intercondylar vertical fracture of tibial plateau; *6*, Condylar fracture of medial or lateral tibia; *7*, Fibular fracture.

are frequently involved in the mechanism of fracture and must always be fully evaluated in determination of the extent of the fracture. Effusion (hemarthrosis) of the knee joint usually is present. Soft tissue must always be considered in prolonged immobilization with fragments in proper alignment because of the possibility of muscular atrophy (quadriceps femorus) and intra-articular adhesions. Improper realignment of the cartilage surface may lead to ultimate arthritic changes (a complication possible even with the best of alignment).

FIGURE 69. Muscular action upon fracture fragments: supracondylar fracture. *Above,* Muscular action about the knee joint. *Below,* Action of the gastrocnemius, pulling the distal fragment posteriorly into the popliteal fossa and the hamstring and quadriceps pulling longitudinally to shorten the femur.
G = Gastrocnemius
H = Hamstrings
Q = Quadriceps

This type of fracture is usually caused by direct violence or torsion stress. Usually there is displacement of the fragments (see Fig. 69) caused by muscular action: the gastrocnemius pulling the distal fragment posteriorly into the fossa and the hamstrings and quadriceps shortening the length of the femur.

Management may be by closed reduction or open reduction, with the former usually possible and desirable. Alignment is attempted on a fracture table and with skeletal traction. If the joint is distended with blood it is aspirated under sterile technique. The hip is flexed (45° to 60°) (Fig. 70). The flexed lower leg tends to reduce the posterior displacement and manual pressure completes this displacement. After reduction a plaster spica is applied with the knee in the flexed position and the wires incorporated into the plaster. Wires are usually removed in 4 to 6 weeks and the cast removed in 6 to 8 weeks.

In cases that defy reduction continuous traction in a Bohler-Braun splint may be necessary. The principles are the same as those just discussed. The gained position of reduction can usually be maintained with 10 to 12 lb. of traction but as much as 20 to 25 lb. of traction for 24 to 48 hours may be necessary. Because muscular atrophy of the quadriceps is early, exercises of the isometric type (quad setting) should be started immediately

FIGURE 70. Management of supracondylar fracture. The hip is flexed 45°. The lower leg, by its weight, reduces the lower femoral fragment assisted by manual pressure, *thick arrow*, upward against the distal fragment. Traction, *TR*, is initially applied to separate the fragments. A spica cast is applied with hip and knee flexed and the pin incorporated.

113

and immobilization in plaster should not be kept any longer than absolutely necessary.

After removal of the spica plaster the leg may be placed in balanced suspension and more active exercises begun. Within 2 to 4 weeks the quadriceps should be reasonably strong and the fracture adequately healed to permit weight-bearing in a walking caliper splint. Obviously time factors are determined by age and severity of fracture as well as patient cooperation.

When close reduction is not possible open reduction may be necessary.

Intercondylar Fractures

These fractures of the femur (Fig. 71) may be of the *Y* or *T* type; they are more severe than supracondylar fractures. Soft tissue injury may be extensive. The fracture may be exceedingly unstable with reduction and maintenance of the reduction difficult.

Management (Fig. 72) is basically that of traction to regain the

FIGURE 71. Intercondylar fractures of the distal femur. *Above left,* Y fracture; *Below right,* T fracture. *Above right* depicts the downward movement of the femur into the intercondylar fracture site separating the two condyles.

length of the femur after aspiration of the joint hemorrhage, manual or clamp manipulation to approximate the condylar fragments, plaster in the reduced position, and *immediate periodic supervised quadriceps exercises*. Postreduction care is similiar to that of supracondylar fracture. Surgical (open) reduction is often necessary to gain proper reduction and to maintain the reduction. The technique will not be detailed. Several types of internal fixation are shown in Figure 73.

Condylar Fractures

Condylar fractures are caused by violence, as are supracondylar and intercondylar, but usually of a different type. Whereas supracondylar and *Y* or *T* intercondylar fractures are often caused by direct linear force, fracture of a condyle occurs from severe varus or valgus force (Fig. 74). The fracture line can be in various planes but usually is vertical and in the sagittal plane. The ligaments of the involved side usually prevent marked displacement but the ligaments of the opposite side and the cruciate ligaments are often damaged.

Management of these fractures depends exclusively on the exact repositioning of the displaced fragment(s) in order to regain continuity of the femoral surface and proper alignment

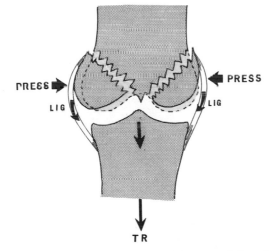

FIGURE 72. Principles of management of intercondylar femoral fracture. Traction, *TR*, elongates the femur by pulling on the collateral ligaments, *LIG*, attached to the condyles, bringing them distally where lateral and medial pressure, *PRESS*, manually or by clamp will approximate the fragments and reduce the fracture in order to allow casting.

with its opposing tibial surface. Closed reduction by traction and manipulation may succeed. Open reduction, using internal fixation of the fragments and repair of the involved ligaments, is often required. Status of the ligaments must be ascertained as well as careful documentation of the exact site and extent of the fractured condyle.

Separation of the Distal Epiphysis

This occurrence may be the result of trauma and will be mentioned only briefly here. The condition occurs usually in boys between the age of 8 to 14 years, usually from direct violence. Several types are shown in Figure 75.

FRACTURES OF PROXIMAL END OF TIBIA

The upper end of the tibia comprises two large condyles separated by a relatively weak bony span (Fig. 76). This fact predisposes the tibial plateau to a high incidence of fractures. The history depicts the exact mechanism of the trauma causing

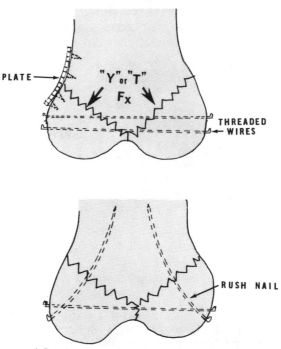

FIGURE 73.   Internal fixation methods of supracondylar fractures of the distal femur.

the fracture, usually direct violence linear to the tibia or violent lateral stresses causing forceful abduction or adduction of the knee. The former is exemplified by landing on one's feet following a hard fall; the latter is exemplified by being struck from the side such as an athletic injury or being hit by a moving vehicle.

FIGURE 74.   Condylar fracture from severe valgus (varus) stress. *Above,* Normal joint anatomy. *Below,* Force applied to the knee joint, T_1, or laterally to the tibia, T_2, can cause fracture of that condyle, *Fx,* tear of the opposite ligament, *LIG,* tear of either or both of the cruciate ligaments, *CRUC,* and compression of the meniscus, *MEN.*

117

The lateral condyle is fractured more frequently than the medial and is associated with injury to the medial ligamentous structures and the cruciate ligaments. The extent of downward and/or lateral displacement is related to the force of the injury. The lateral meniscus may be crushed, forced within the com-

FIGURE 75. Separation of the distal epiphysis. The epiphysis can be separated dependent on the direction of the force. *A*, The normal epiphysis; *B*, The epiphysis is tilted forward; *C*, The rarer type in which the epiphysis is tilted backward; *D*, The epiphysis may be displaced medially or laterally also.

minution, or forced into the knee joint medially (Fig. 77). Severe adduction force upon the tibia (lateral force upon the knee joint) may cause fracture of the medial condyle, tear of the lateral collateral ligaments, and crushing of the medial meniscus.

Direct violence, such as a fall on extended legs, can cause vertical fracture of the tibial plateau in a *Y* or *T* fracture (Fig. 78). The ligaments may remain intact or be individually or singly injured. The center fragment may project into the fracture site and cause varying degrees of deformity. Effusion of the joint with blood is usual as these fractures are intra-articular in nature.

Management demands complete evaluation of the mechanism of fracture, relationship of the residual fragments, ligamentous injury, and the sequelae of soft tissue injuries. The aim of treatment is to restore the articular surfaces to their anatomical relationships, i.e. restoration of the tibial plateau articular surface, proper relationship to the femoral condyles, restoration of ligamentous integrity, evacuation of any intra-articular debris, and restoration of quadriceps strength.

Management of fracture of the lateral tibial condyle begins with aspiration of hemarthrosis. If there is no displacement start active quadriceps exercises after application of a snugfitting *un padded* plaster cast with knee in full extension. In two weeks a new plaster is applied that remains an additional two weeks

FIGURE 76. Tibial condyles: stress plates. The upper end of the tibia is comprised of two condyles: strong cortical bone, *S*, separated by a weaker bone span, *W*.

119

when flexion exercises are begun. Weight bearing is usually permitted in 10 to 12 weeks although crutch ambulation without weight bearing is started much sooner.

If the lateral fragment is separated and depressed after the joint is aspirated, traction along the line of the tibia is applied (Fig. 79) with simultaneous lateral traction applied by a large bandage passing about the medial aspect of the knee to cause varus of the knee. This last maneuver causes the lateral collateral ligament to pull up on the tibial fragment and reduce the separation. Direct pressure by the surgeon on the fragment will

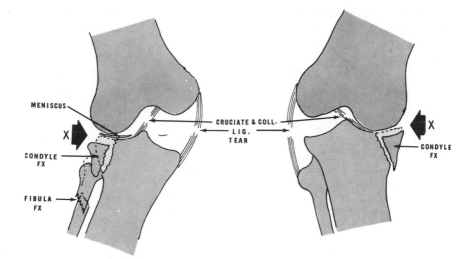

FIGURE 77. Fracture of the lateral tibial condyle. Lateral stress or uneven direct force can cause depressed fracture of the lateral condyle, crushed lateral meniscus, tear of cruciate ligaments, and tear of the medial collateral ligaments.

FIGURE 78. Direct trauma to the tibial plateau. Direct trauma, such as a fall on extended legs, can cause a Y or T fracture of the plateau.

120

further reduce the depression. A compression clamp may be used by an experienced surgeon. Medial depressed tibial fractures are treated in a similar manner with the forces applied in the opposite transverse direction to cause knee *valgus*.

After reduction the leg is casted and exercises begun as stated. The cast is kept on for 8 weeks with weight bearing possible in 10 to 12 weeks, preferably *without* a knee brace if the quadriceps are sufficiently strong.

In a severely comminuted fracture the fragments may be avascular and result in asceptic necrosis. The fragments may wedge the separated fragments and prevent close opposition. If the fragments remain separated and the surface margin irregular, degenerative arthritis, far more severe than normally expected, may result. Tears in the cartilage become filled with

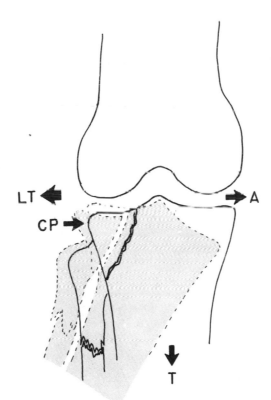

FIGURE 79. Principles of treatment of tibial plateau fracture. *A*, Aspirate the hemarthrosis or effusion; *T*, Apply traction; *LT*, Apply lateral traction to cause varus and open the lateral aspect of the joint; *CP*, Compression against fragment to reduce fracture, which can be done manually or with a clamp. Cast with snug plaster.

fibrous tissue and may create an adequate weight-bearing surface with full range of motion.

If immediate reduction is not attainable prolonged traction in a Bohler-Braun splint using 10 to 12 lb. of traction may be beneficial for reduction. If closed reduction is not possible open reduction with internal fixation after reduction may be necessary. These indications and techniques are well documented in orthopedic literature.

FRACTURES OF THE PATELLA

Fracture of the patella has been discussed in detail in Chapter 5. Please refer to that section of text.

BIBLIOGRAPHY

Olerud, S.: Operative treatment of supracondylar-condylar fractures of the femur. J. Bone Joint Surg. [Am] 54:1015, 1972.

CHAPTER 8

Congenital and Acquired Deformities of the Knee

The term "congenital" implies its presence at or before birth and such deformities are common in the musculoskeletal system. They may be grouped into various categories:

1. Failure of tissue differentiation such as failure of cartilage to progress into bone.
2. Failure of fusion as exemplified in bipartite patella
3. Supernumerary parts.
4. Deformity in the bone itself such as osteogenesis imperfecta or congenital bowing.

Bone dysplasia is considered to be a congenital variance as well as being biochemical, hormonal, and metabolic. These dystrophies and dysplasias are well documented (Stelling and Rubin). Most are rare and few affect the knee singly, but in the generalized involvement of the child the knee may also be included. *Dysplasia* (Rubin) is described as a disturbance in bone development and is *intrinsic* to bone. *Dystrophy* is defective bone development caused by *extrinsic* factors such as metabolic or nutritional abnormalities. *Dysostosis* is abnormal bone development caused by a *defect* in ectodermal or mesenchymal tissues.

In all three conditions the extremities usually are deformed and shortened, and cause abnormal gait. The knee, besides involvement in length of the extremity, may be varus or valgus.

Genu valgum, genu varum, genu recurvatum, and tibial or femoral torsion are the most frequent deformities noted in childhood that cause parental concern over abnormal gait. Although they ususally are congenital or familial they may be acquired following injury or disease or may be secondary to systemic disease.

123

Genu valgum is an angular deformity of the leg, otherwise termed knock-knee, in which the ankles are separated when the knees are in contact (Fig. 80). This condition is frequently noted in childhood and there is a large familial tendency. It is often associated with severely pronated feet and in overweight children who begin ambulation at an early age. It may be secondary to rickets or fractures of the femur; caused by trauma to the epiphyseal plate, paralysis by lower motor neuron disease, cerebral palsy, or a hip defect; or idiopathic. It is frequently noted from age two to six and is of concern when it persists to a significant degree after that age.

Prognosis depends on the etiological factors. When the malleoli are less than three inches apart conservative treatment or natural development usually ends in good results. Conservative treatment consists of correcting the foot pronation with an inner wedge of a stiff one-eighth inch counter in shoes, weight loss, and passive stretching exercises administered by the parents.

In a severe genu valgus, surgery consists of stapling or osteotomy planned carefully depending upon the age of the child, the severity of the deformity, and the calculated growth potential (Fig. 81).

 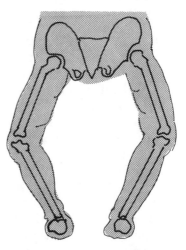

VALGUS   VARUS

FIGURE 80. Genu valgus and genu varus. *Left,* Genu valgus with the knees close to each other and the ankles separated. *Right,* Genu varus showing knees separated and ankles together.

GENU VARUM

Genu varum is an alignment abnormality of the leg in which the knees are widely separated while the ankle malleoli are in contact. This condition is commonly called bowlegs.

All normal babies at birth and during infancy have some degree of genu varum. The condition frequently persists during the first three years. Much of the varus is apparent rather than actual as a result of the normal distribution of thigh fat, the position of the legs caused by the interposition of thick diapers,

FIGURE 81. Surgical treatment of valgus or varus. *1*, The knee joint in genu valgus with the open epiphyseal line of the distal femur and proximal tibia. *2*, Stapling in which the growth on the convex side is stopped, permitting continued growth on the other side, *arrows*, with stapling held until alignment is achieved. *3*, Osteotomy of the tibia in which a wedge is removed to permit the distal portion's being brought under the proximal portion and the leg realigned.

and early weight bearing in chubby children. The condition is aggravated by the coexistence of tibial torsion. Physiological bowing is symmetrical and involves both femur and tibia; x-ray views show cortical thickening of the medial side of the bones (Fig. 82). Although most genu varum is physiologically caused it may be the result of vitamin D deficiency from renal rickets or resistant dietary rickets, osteochondritis (Blount's disease), dyschondroplasia, osteogenesis imperfecta, epiphyseal injury, or neurofibromatosis.

FIGURE 82. X-ray evidence of cortical thickening in valgus. It is on the concave side as a result of stress of weight bearing.

Proper diagnosis is mandatory for proper treatment, but certain principles affect the results of any treatment. It is usually desirable to avoid precipitous early walking, insure proper bed position during sleeping, avoid excessive diapering, and institute gentle manipulative exercises by the parents. Braces are advocated for the moderate deformity that persists in later child-

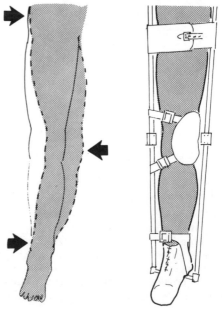

FIGURE 83. Brace treatment of valgus. A long leg brace can be constructed, which places three points of pressure, *arrows*, to correct valgus (or varus in reversed manner).

hood (Fig. 83) or when very severe surgical intervention may be required such as stapling procedures or osteotomy. If the child is walking a shoe correction aids in realigning the superincumbent leg. In varus an outer wedge on the shoe of one-eighth to one-fourth inch is prescribed (Fig. 84). The efficacy of this is not confirmed.

TIBIAL TORSION

This condition may coexist with genu varus and genu valgus or be present alone. Tibial torsion in children designates torsion (twist) in the bone (tibia) in the coronal plane causing the medial malleolus to lie in a different plane than the lateral malleolus. If there is internal torsion the medial malleolus is behind the lateral. This condition exists in the fetus but at birth the malleoli are equal. By walking age, 20° of external rotation is considered normal. More recent studies (Khermosh) indicate that newborns have external rotation of 2.2° with gradual external torsion angle of 1.3° per year. Many investigators and clinicians deny the presence of tibial torsion in either direction. Most often tibial torsion is a self-limiting physiological condition and may be a result of internal or external rotation of the hip. Internal tibial torsion is frequently associated with bowing, metatarsus varus, or talipes equinovarus (clubfoot). External rotation is often associated with knock-knee deformity.

If mild and not of significant cosmetic concern no treatment is needed. Functional impairment at the worst is an abnormal gait and, in childhood, tripping over one's own feet. Treatment consists of manipulative exercises done by the parents and shoe corrections to build up the inner or outer aspect of the sole and/or heel to cause either inversion or eversion as the condition dictates. Denis-Browne splints are advocated by some but considered useless and unphysiological by others in so far as the stress of the splint seems to be expended to rotate the knee and not the tibial torsion (Fig. 85). Twisters may be prescribed but their value is questionable. The likelihood of their correcting torsion is limited and there is the possibility that twisters may create or aggravate knee valgus as a result of their stress (Fig. 86).

TIBIAL VARUM

Angular deformities can occur in any plane but the majority are in the coronal (valgus or varus) or in the sagittal plane

127

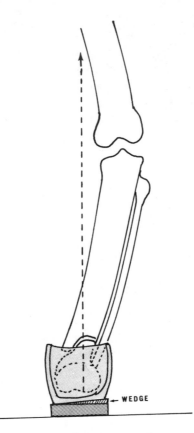

FIGURE 84.   Shoe wedge treatment of genu varus. In an attempt to realign the weight-bearing stress on the knee a sole and heel wedge may be prescribed for the outer border of the shoe. The efficacy of this is not confirmed.

DENIS – BROWNE SPLINT

FIGURE 85.   Denis-Browne night splints. The Denis-Browne splint is a pair of shoes for varus or valgus of the foot. The shoes are separated in specific degree of rotation by bending the bar. The length of the bar is equal to the desired separation of the legs as is the degeee of external rotation. The bar places rotatory stress at the knee and may not be influential upon the tibial torsion.

(recurvatum). A form of tibia varum resulting from osteochondrosis (osteochondrosis deformans tibia or Blount's disease) requires separate discussion from the so-called physiological bowing. In osteochondrosis deformans there is disturbance of growth involving the metaphysis epiphysial cartilage and the osseous center of the epiphysis. The pathological conditions are located on the medial side of the proximal tibial epiphysis causing an abrupt varus angular deformity (Fig. 87). The condition may be unilateral but 50 per cent of the cases are bilateral.

The criteria of osteochondrosis tibia varum are

1. A sharp angular deformity immediately below the proximal tibial epiphysis.
2. An irregular epiphysial cartilage.
3. A wedge-shaped osseous portion of the epiphysis.
4. A beak projection forming from the medial metaphysis.
5. Lax medial ligaments.

Onset usually is insidious. If bilateral, the child develops a

"TWISTERS"

FIGURE 86.   Twister braces. Attached to a pelvic band and fixed to the shoe, the twister brace is a set of bilateral spring cables in a housing that tends to externally rotate the leg. The main value of this brace appears to be in the training of inversion gait towards more external rotation. Its static correction is doubtful.

waddle gait; if the condition is unilateral the child develops a limp. Clinically the leg reveals a sharp angular deformity below the knee. Treatment is expectant and conservative because spontaneous correction does occur. Since this deformity does not progress after the epiphysis (cartilage) is closed, operative intervention for correction probably should be deferred until closure is ascertained.

GENU RECURVATUM

Genu recurvatum has numerous causes ranging from intrinsic pathological conditions of the knee to secondary factors. The most common cause is fixed plantar flexion from either contracture (of numerous etiologies) or spastic equinus. Excessive compensation of the quadriceps plus weak gastrocnemius soleus may be causative. (See Chapter 9 on gait for explanation.) Ex-

FIGURE 87.   Osteochondrosis deformans tibia: Blount's disease. This entity, described by W. Blount, is medial osteochondrosis with sharp angular deformity immediately below the proximal tibial epiphysis, an irregular medial cartilage, the medial metaphysis forming a beak-like projection, *P*, and lax medial ligaments, *L*.

FIGURE 88.   Treatment of genu recurvatum by short leg brace. A brace with a down-stop at the ankle. By decreasing equinus and thus secondary back knee, it may be effective in preventing recurvatum. *C*, Mechanical principle of the brace: *S*, the stop; *CP*, calf pressure; *curved arrow*, the allowable excursion of the upright bars of the brace on the fixed foot to the floor.

FIGURE 89.   Back heel brace for genu recurvatum. *A*, The usual back knee stance, regardless of numerous etiological factors. *B*, Brace designed to control recurvatum in standing and permits sitting, *C. D*, The brace is a dynamic splint made of orthoplast with 25° flexion molded into splint. (Cf: Andersen in Bibliography.)

131

cessive gluteal contractions with no soleus or quadriceps may also cause recurvatum.

Treatment is based on correction of the etiological factor(s) and may consist of exercises to regain muscle balance or to stretch the offending contracture. Serial casts may be applied. It is important to consider surgical release of the offending muscle-tendons *before* excessive changes occur. A brace with an ankle down-stop may be useful (Fig. 88); this may be incorporated with a back knee stop that simultaneously permits knee flexion for walking and sitting. The knee portion of the brace that prevents back knee also applies pressure to aid proprioception at the pressure sites (Fig. 89).

BIBLIOGRAPHY

Andersen, C. B.: Dynamic knee splint to prevent hyperextension. Phys. Ther. 52:944, 1972.

Blount, W. P.: Tibia vara. J. Bone Joint Surg. 19:1, 1937.

Hutter, C. G., and Scott, W.: Tibial torsion. J. Bone Joint Surg. [Am] 31:511, 1949.

Khermosh, O., Lior, G., and Weissman, S. L.: Tibial torsion in children. Clin. Orthop. 79:25, 1971.

Kleven, D. K., Perry, J., and Hislop, H.: The ankle joint: An anatomical and mechanical study using amputated specimens. Thesis. Los Angeles, 1970.

Majestro, T. C., and Frost, H. M.: Posterior transposition of the origins of the anatomic internal rotators of the hip. Clin. Orthop. 79:57, 1971.

Perry, J.: Bracing the knee. J. Canad. Physiotherap. Assoc. 24:198, 1972.

Rubin, P.: Dynamic Classification of Bone Dysplasia. New Year Book Medical Publishers, Chicago, 1964.

Smith, E. M., and Juvinall, R. R.: Mechanics of bracing, in Licht, Sidney (ed.): Orthotics Etcetera. Licht, New Haven, 1966.

Stelling, F. H.: General affection of the skeletal system. Pediatr. Clin. North Am. 14:359, 1967.

CHAPTER 9

The Knee in Gait:
Normal and Abnormal

The functional knee in stance and in gait in childhood and adulthood must be understood before specifics of the abnormal gait and stance can be evaluated and remedied. Factors to be considered are (1) quadriceps competency, (2) neuromuscular incoordination, (3) limitation of range of motion, (4) proprioception adequacy, and (5) relationship and adequacy of contiguous joints (the hip and/or ankle). All must be taken into consideration in evaluating proper knee function or its relative dysfunction.

In the normal gait the trunk shifts from side to side with approximately 2 cm. of displacement. This motion attempts to minimize vertical body displacement to decrease energy expenditure. This trunk shift, laterally and rotatory, requires precise external muscular control and delicate proprioception. The total body weight above the pelvis consists of: trunk, 50 percent of total body weight; head, 8 percent; each upper extremity, 8 percent; and during the swing phase the swinging leg, 15 percent. At the one leg stance during gait 85 percent of the total body weight must be balanced.

At heel strike the hip extensors bring the body forward above the weight-bearing leg (Fig. 90). The knee of the striking leg maintains a slight knee flexion (10° to 15°) to dampen the impact. If there is hip extensor weakness the pelvis moves ahead (further) over the center of gravity and further flexes the knee (see Fig. 90), which causes the femur to be more horizontal and thus creates more stress upon the weight-bearing quadriceps. Good hip extensors and good proprioceptive sense will extend the hip and pull the thigh over the fixed lower leg and foot and thus impose less stress upon the quadriceps. During this gait

133

phase (heel strike to stance phase) over the fixed foot, the lower leg must achieve stability with adequate ankle plantar flexors.

A weak soleus, or a gait in which the soleus for push-off is not effective, permits the knee to flex during the stance gait (Fig. 91). In a foot that has a contracted soleus group (contracture or neurological spasticity) the plantar flexed (fixed) foot me-

FIGURE 90. Gait analysis. *A*, Normal gait with heel strike, *HS*, the knee slightly flexed to dampen the impact. The hip extensors, *G*, extend the hip and pull the pelvis over the weight-bearing leg at the stance phase. *B*, Gait with weak gluteal (hip) extensors, *G*, that fail to extend the hip, and thus at stance phase the knee is still flexed as the pelvis passes over the fixed foot. *Right,* The foot is in equinus stance and is not related to the hip weakness.

FIGURE 91. Effect of weak soleus gait on the knee. *1,* The anticus (ankle dorsiflexor), *An,* at heel strike prevents foot slap. *2,* As the pelvis passes over the fixed foot during stance phase the gastrocnemius-soleus muscle, *G,* prevents excessive ankle dorsiflexion and decelerates the leg as it passes over the fixed foot. This action simultaneously prevents the knee from flexing in stance, *3,* With a weak soleus, *G,* excessive ankle dorsiflexion occurs and the knee flexes unless strong quadriceps and/or strong hip extensors intervene.

chanically extends the knee as the pelvis passes over the center of gravity (Fig. 92). Contracture of the posterior knee tissues, causing a flexed knee, places excessive stress upon the quadriceps and can be assisted by strong hip extensor and ankle plantar flexor groups. Fifteen degrees of flexion can be accepted if the ankle and hip musculature is strong enough to compensate for the flexure (Fig. 93). A hip flexion contracture also flexes the weight-bearing knee and can be balanced by adequate quadriceps and soleus. The forward flexed posture, where the upper body brings the center of gravity ahead of the knee (see Fig. 93), places stress on all the leg extensors.

A patient with weak knee extensors (quadriceps) *and* weak hip extensors can lean backwards with his trunk in order to balance over his center of gravity. This requires good proprioception and muscle control.

Weak ankle plantar flexors can cause knee instability since the quadriceps do not contract quickly enough to prevent tripping or knee buckling. Loss of proprioception also can contribute to the condition. A short leg brace that controls plantar *or* dorsiflexion may be needed to improve gait. The type of brace is determined by careful gait analysis.

Patients suffering from flaccid paralysis (peripheral neuropathy, amyotrophic lateral sclerosis, polio, etc.) who have good

FIGURE 92. Equinus gait: contracted or spastic soleus. *A*, There is no heel strike because the foot is in equinus during the swing phase. *B*, Normally extended knee. As the pelvis passes over the fixed foot the shortened soleus extends the knee mechanically. If the equinus is excessive, *B₁*, back knee (hyperextension) can occur, *broken line*. *C*, In a marked equinus during the last part of the stance phase the foot can rock over the weight-bearing toes and throw the pelvis ahead of the center of gravity. This imposes marked stress upon the quadriceps or permits falling if the quads are inadequate.

proprioception can accomodate well to their paresis. With impaired proprioception such as in myelomeningoceles or with poor motor control as in cerebral palsy and stroke, compensatory gait is difficult to achieve. Children with myelomeningocele usually lack strong gastrocnemius-soleus muscles as well as hip extensors *and* have impaired sensory level. Loss of proprioception or loss of motor control may be an indication for bracing.

CONCLUSION

Careful evaluation of the function or malfunction of the knee requires

1. Neurological examination for motor, spastic, or flaccid paresis and proprioception.

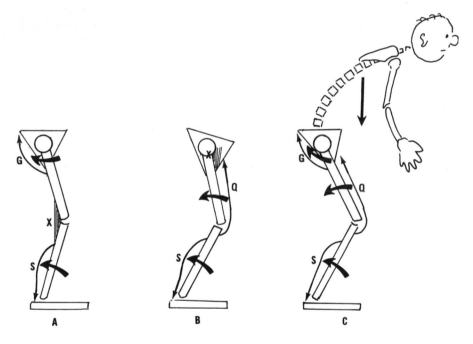

FIGURE 93. Pathological stance phase of gait. *A*, Flexed knee stance caused by contracture, *X*, of the knee. Erect stance is possible with strong hip extensors (*G*, gluteals) and strong plantar flexors (*S*, soleus). *B*, Flexed stance as a result of hip flexion contracture, *X*, overcome by strong quadriceps, *Q*, and strong soleus, *S*. The former extends the knee and the latter pulls the leg back over the fixed foot. *C*, Flexed stance resulting from bent-over posture with most of the body weight (60 to 65%) placed ahead of the center of gravity. All extensors are needed to maintain erect stance.

2. Orthopedic evaluation for contracture or malalignment.
3. Careful stance and gait evaluation.

Upon performance of all these tests and careful evaluation of their significance proper treatment can be prescribed: be it exercise, bracing, or surgery. Failure of definitive treatment can be related to improper evaluation more often than to faulty treatment technique.

BIBLIOGRAPHY

Basmajian, J. V.: Muscles Alive. Their Function Revealed by Electromyography. Williams & Wilkins Baltimore, 1962.

Levens, A. S., Inman, V. T., and Blosser, J. A.: Transverse rotation of the segments of the lower extremity in locomotion. J. Bone Joint Surg. [Am] 30:859, 1948.

Liberson, W. T.: Biomechanics of gait: A method of study. Arch Phys. Med. Rehabil., 46:37, 1965.

Murray, M. P., Drought, A. B., and Kory, R. C.: Walking patterns of normal men. J. Bone Joint Surg. [Am] 46:335, 1964.

Perry, J.: Bracing of the knee. J. Can. Physiother. Assoc. 24:298, 1972.

Saunders, J. B. de C. M., Inman, V. T., and Eberhart, H. D.: Major determinants in normal and pathological gait. J. Bone Joint Surg. [Am] 35:543, 1953.

Schenker, A. W.: Pathological implications of abnormal stance and gait. Occup. Ther. and Rehabil. 28:131, 1949.

CHAPTER 10

The Knee in Cerebral Palsy

The knee is involved in most types of cerebral palsy as a result of muscle imbalance or secondary to hip or foot-ankle deviation, contracture, or surgical intervention. The goals of treatment of cerebral palsy are to develop and utilize to potential that which is not present as a result of central nervous system damage before, at, or after birth. Treatment is thus to correct defect when possible, prevent new defects that may occur, improve the remaining capacities, and prevent unwanted substitutions but simultaneously provide and encourage desirable substitution functions.

The child with a birth defect of the central nervous system may be born with a specific type of defect but this defect or its disability may change during the subsequent stages of development from early weeks of life. The exact type of defect and its resultant disability often varies with each examination.

Ambulation receives priority in considering the evaluation and stress of treatment. Hand dexterity and communication *should* receive priority but ambulation is demanded of the parents. Numerous forms of treatment have had their claimants in the treatment of cerebral palsy: intracranial cortical surgical ablation, cranial blood vessel ligation, cord tracheotomies, ventral root or dorsal root surgery, and alcohol or phenol nerve blocks to alter the neuromuscular abnormality, imbalance, or incoordination. No surgical procedure, be it upon the central nervous system, peripheral nervous system, or any aspect of the musculoskeletal system, alters the underlying abnormal pattern(s) of movement. The main benefit of surgical procedure is prevention or alteration of deformity and improvement of function and/or appearance.

Treatment by exercise aims to improve strength, balance, and coordination and increase range of articular motion. In cerebral palsy, classification of the hypotonic or athetoid child is not of concern regarding joint limitation, but this is a concern in the spastic or tension patient. In this latter category the concern is more of contracture of the legs in the hip flexors and/or adductors, hamstrings, and the gastrocnemius-soleus muscle groups. Exercises to stretch these groups, when instituted early, persistently, and correctly, may be effective. If all these criteria are met and, with combined proper use of splinting, the limitation persists or progresses, surgical intervention, such as muscle-tendon transplantation and/or release should be given serious consideration.

Exercises obviously are limited in their application as to duration, intensity, frequency, and tolerance by the patient and the therapist or parents. Properly prescribed and fitted night splints or braces will have definite value to maintain the gains made by judicious daytime exercises. At the present time drugs given parenterally or orally have proven disappointing.

Evaluation of the cerebral palsied patient may mislead the unwary or unskilled examiner in the interpretation of weakness of specific muscle groups with inadequate function when the weakness is essentially comparative weakness of agonist pitted against an unyielding overwhelming spastic antagonist. Release of this opposing antagonist may often restrengthen the alleged weak ineffectual agonist and functional improvement may result.

The child with cerebral palsy must first develop head and neck balance before any further antigravity function can be expected. This must be followed by improved trunk control used in sitting balance. Hand and arm function are required before the next stage, standing balance, can be sought and achieved. Gait evolves after standing balance by acquiring strength, agonist-antagonist balance, and reciprocal movement.

Numerous techniques of physiotherapy are availabe to train the child in better neck and head balance, sitting trunk balance, and standing balance. Standing balance is aided by support within a mechanical apparatus that encircles the patient. This is followed by support from a wall behind the child; from which he gradually progresses to unassisted balance. At first stance is begun with wide based footing while standing between parallel bars. The child progresses to canes with a wide base (weighted or not, as indicated) and then gait training. The use of a walker delays development of balance. Excessive bracing that denies all undesired motions is also questioned and probably better avoided. Each stage of function and each stage of development must be reevaluated. The treatment of the neuromuscularly defective child is not static and each stage must be ascertained.

Since the subject of this book is the knee this specific joint must be evaluated although the remainder of the child must not be ignored. Knee function depends upon stress factors imparted upon it by the foot-ankle position, balance of the tonus of the opposing flexors and extensors, contracture of the periarticular soft tissues, and coordinated neuromuscular action of all the muscles about the knee, the foot-ankle, the hip, and the superincumbent trunk.

In athetosis, which constitutes 25 percent of cerebral palsy cases, braces may be used in the lower extremity essentially for *training*, not for correction or prevention of contracture. Braces are of no value in the ataxic form of cerebral palsy; in this condition skis, weighted shoes, square heels on the shoes, and physiotherapy exercises are of value. Braces applied to the lower extremity may be used to direct specific motion and prevent unwanted motion but their value in this approach is questioned by many physicians.

A deforming condition which occurs in the spastic type of cerebral palsy is spastic internal femoral torsion. This consists of internal rotation of the distal femur in relation to the proximal femur. Clinically, although the patella points straight ahead when the patient is standing or lying supine, the patella points (rotates) inward when the patient walks. This is frequently concomitant with associated internal tibial torsion, compensatory external tibial torsion, or genu valgum that allow the feet to point directly ahead during gait. Internal femoral torsion owing to spasticity appears when the child begins walking at age 1.5 to 2.0 years and becomes stable at maturity with no further progression.

Related etiologically to spastic internal femoral torsion is adductor spasticity with the child becoming erect in a spastic crouch posture. The adductors are not *normally* internal rotators but when the knees are held in the flexed position as in the crouch posture and the foot *fixed* to the floor (weight-bearing) the adductors become internal rotators (Fig. 94).

In the crouch posture during gait at heel-strike there is an adductor twist which simulates internal rotation. If this condition is bilateral a scissoring gait results. In this gait owing to spasticity, at heel strike the tensor fascia femoris and the gluteus minimus *overcontract* and add to internal rotation of the hip.

The commonly used twister brace (see Fig. 86) to eliminate

internal rotation during gait may aggravate the rotation and intensify the valgus knee posture with minimal temporary benefit and *no* permanent recovery. Treatment is best initiated by adductor tenotomy and neurectomy of the anterior branch of the obturator nerve done *extrapelvicly.* If the internal rotation and scissoring is severe consideration must be given to stripping the origin of the tensor fascia femoris and the gluteus minimus, which now, in the crouch posture, are functionally internal rotators. The procedure is to roll posteriorly the anterior origin from the iliac crest and bifurcate it to the capsule of the hip capsule. By this posterior move the line of pull is that of *external* rotation, at least removing its *internal* rotatory pull.

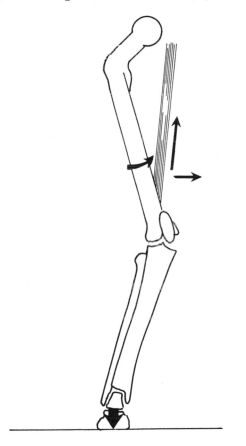

FIGURE 94. Internal femoral torsion from adductor mechanism. When the foot is fixed to the floor, *arrow,* and the knee and hip flexed in the crouch position of cerebral palsy, the adductors that act upon the leg cause valgus at the knee and internally rotate the femur. If this occurs bilaterally the classic scissor gait results.

There are several basic indications of surgery (Eggers):

1. Elimination or diminution of an unwanted muscle function by procedures such as neurectomy.
2. Alteration of function of a muscle group such as causing a flexor to become an extensor.
3. Negation by moving *part* of a muscle to cause a *biarthrodal* muscle to become a *monoarthrodal* muscle (for instance the recession of the gastrocnemius that acts across the posterior knee joint and inserting it below, thus causing its action merely at the ankle joint).
4. A negative-positive alteration, which is similiar to negation, in order to transfer the hamstrings from the tibia to attach to the femur and thus decrease knee flexion (negative), improve hip extension (positive), and incidentally improve hip adduction and decrease lumbar lordosis (Fig. 95).

There are modifications to Eggers' classic procedure, depen-

"CROUCH"

FIGURE 95. Crouch position in spastic cerebral palsy: Eggers' procedure. *Left,* Crouch posture caused by spastic hamstrings, *H,* flexing the knee. There is a simultaneous hip flexion and foot equinus. *Right,* By transplanting the hamstring insertions from the tibia to the posterior femur, knee flexion is eliminated. The hips thus extend more and the equinus is improved or corrected.

142

dent upon the desired result, the extent of desired correction of deforming muscle forces, and the anticipated resultant function for that particular patient. If ambulation is not anticipated, all hamstring muscles are divided to minimize flexion contracture and the resultant nursing and child care needs. If the child walks with a crouch gait but has full knee extension when recumbent the Egger's procedure merely divides the gracilis, lengthens the semimembranosus, and transfers the semitendinosus and the biceps. If ankle equinus persists after hamstring transfer a neurectomy of the soleus or a tendoachilles lengthening may need to be considered. The need, the extent, and the type of procedure indicated are decided with careful evaluation.

Treatment of cerebral palsy by nonsurgical measures is varied with numerous techniques, principals, methods, and equivocal results. Exercises are varied, including those intended to maintain full range of motion by passive stretching, balance the agonist with the spastic antagonists, re-educate the central nervous system by proprioceptive techniques, inhibit reflexes, utilize pathological reflexes, and stimulate cutaneous and musculocutaneous reflexes. The basis of some of these techniques can be gleaned from the bibliography.

BIBLIOGRAPHY

Bobath, K., and Bobath, B. A.: A treatment of cerebral palsy. Brit. J. Phys. Med. 15:105, 1952.

Cailliet, R.: Bracing for Spasticity, in Licht, Sidney (ed.): Orthotics Etcetera. Licht, New Haven, 1966.

Deaver, G. G.: Methods of treating the neuromuscular disabilities. Arch. Phys. Med. Rehabil. 37:363, 1956.

Eggers, G. W. N.: Transplantation of hamstring tendons to femoral condyles in order to improve hip extension and to decrease knee flexion in cerebral spastic paralysis. J. Bone Joint Surg. [Am] 34:827, 1952.

Eggers, G. W. N.: Surgical division of the patella retinacula to improve extension of the knee joint in cerebral spastic paralysis. J. Bone Joint Surg. [Am] 32:80, 1950.

Eggers, G. W. N., and Evans, E. B.: Surgery in cerebral palsy. A.A.O.S. instructional course lecture. J. Bone Joint Surg. [Am] 45:1275, 1963.

Fay, T.: The use of pathological and unlocking reflexes in the rehabilitation of spastics. Am. J. Phys. Med. 33:347, 1954.

Gillette, H. E.: Kinesiology of cerebral palsy. Clin. Orthop. 47:31, 1966.

Kabat, H.: Studies on neuromuscular dysfunction. XI. New principals of neuromuscular reeducation. Permant. Found. Med. Bull. 5:3, 1947.

Knott, M., and Voss, D. E.: Proprioceptive Neuromuscular Facilitation, ed. 2. Harper & Row, New York, 1968.

Majestro, T. C., and Frost, H. M.: Cerebral palsy: Spastic internal femoral torsion. Clin. Orthop. 79:44, 1971.

143

Index

144

145

146

Meniscectomy, 44
Meniscus (Menisci), 5-6
  bursitis and, 108
  disease of, 75
  flexion-extension and, 37, 41-42
  fractures and, 118
  injuries of, 40-60
  rotation and, 37
Metatarsus varus, tibial torsion and, 127
Motion, 1, 33. *See also* Extension; Flexion; Rotation.
Motor neuron disease, genu valgum and, 124
Mucopolysaccharides, 98, 102
Muscle(s), 16-29
  atrophy of, 90, 112, 113
  during extension, 39
  importance of, 8
  inadequacy of, 43
Myositis ossificans, 71

NAILING, 83
Nerve
  femoral, damage to, 103
  injury to, ligamentous injuries and, 67
  peroneal, subluxation and, 68
  sciatic, 27
Nerve supply, 16, 27
Neurectomy, 141
Neurofibromatosis, 126
Night braces, 139

OBESITY, 43, 69, 75, 106, 124
Osgood-Schlatter's disease, 80-81
Ossification, 1-4, 83
Osteoarthritis, 47, 90, 97-99, 106
Osteoarthrosis, 47, 90, 97-99, 106
Osteochondral fractures, 76-77
Osteochondritis, 80-81, 83, 127
Osteochondritis dissecans, 81-83
Osteochondrosis, 129
Osteoporosis, 79
Osteotomy, 95, 99, 124, 127

PAIN, 44
  arthritis and, 90, 97
  bursitis and, 107
  capsular or ligamentous injury and, 47, 63
  fear of, 93
  fractures and, 110

  in differential diagnosis, 30
  low threshold of, 93
  meniscus injuries and, 44
  patellar problems and, 75, 77, 79, 80, 81
  tendon and, 70
Pannus, 86-88, 92, 105
Paralysis, 124, 135
Patella, 1, 16
  during extension, 38-39
  fracture of, 75-77, 122
  injury and diseases of, 73-84
Patellectomy, 80
Phenylbutazone, 92
Plasma in hemophilic arthritis, 100
Popliteal cysts, 108
Popliteus muscle, 29, 33
Posterior bursitis, 108
Postoperative rehabilitation program in meniscus injuries, 55
Power vs. endurance in exercises, 55-60
P. R. E., 58-60
Progressive resistance exercise, 56, 58-60
Proprioception, 135, 136
Prostheses, 95
Proteolytic enzyme, 98
PTC level, 102
Pulley vs. weight, 61
Pyogenic arthritis, 106-107

QUADRICEPS exercises, 55-59, 80, 104, 115, 119
Quadriceps femoris muscle, 16
Quadriceps femoris tendon, 16
Quadriceps mechanism
  atrophy of, 45, 92, 112, 113
  paralysis of, 103-104
  rupture of, 68-71

REDUCTION
  fractures and, 113, 116, 121, 122
  meniscus injuries and, 52-53
Resistive exercises, 56, 57, 58-59, 93, 103
Rheumatoid arthritis, 85-96
  differential diagnosis in, 97, 106
Rickets, 124, 126
R.M., 58-60
Rotation, 19, 25, 33-39, 40, 41
  in clinical meniscus signs, 47
  prevention of, 9

147

148

Weight reduction in osteoarthritis, 98
Weight vs. pulley, 60
Weighted shoes, 140
Wrisberg, ligament of, 6

X-RAY studies
  arthritis and, 91-92, 100, 106
  fractures and, 75, 76, 77, 110
  genu varum and, 126
  myositis ossificans and, 71

neoplasms and, 107
patellar problems and, 75, 76, 79, 80, 81, 83
severe sprain and, 65

Y LIGAMENT of Bigelow, 29
Young. *See also* Teenagers.
  chondromalacia patellae and, 77
  injury of quadriceps mechanism in, 68, 70